9762588

# Groupwork with Women/ Groupwork with Men

## An Overview of Gender Issues in Social Groupwork Practice

The *Social Work with Groups* series

Series Editors: Catherine P. Papell and Beulah Rothman

- *Co-Leadership in Social Work with Groups,* Catherine P. Papell and Beulah Rothman

- *Social Groupwork & Alcoholism,* Marjorie Altman and Ruth Crocker, Guest Editors

- *Group Work with the Frail Elderly,* Shura Saul, Guest Editor

- *The Use of Group Services in Permanency Planning for Children,* Sylvia Morris, Guest Editor

- *Activities and Action in Groupwork,* Ruth Middleman, Guest Editor

- *Groupwork with Women/Groupwork with Men: An Overview of Gender Issues in Social Groupwork Practice,* Beth Glover Reed and Charles D. Garvin, Guest Editors

- *Ethnicity in Groupwork Practice,* Larry Davis, Guest Editor

- *Time as a Factor in Groupwork,* Albert Alissi and Max Casper, Guest Editors

- *Groupwork with Children & Adolescents,* Ralph Kolodny and James Garland, Guest Editors

- *William Schwartz Memorial Issue* (title to be announced), Alex Gitterman and Lawrence Shulman, Guest Editors

# Groupwork with Women/ Groupwork with Men

## An Overview of Gender Issues in Social Groupwork Practice

Beth Glover Reed and Charles D. Garvin
Guest Editors

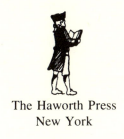

The Haworth Press
New York

HV
45
G735
1983

*Groupwork with Women/Groupwork with Men: An Overview of Gender Issues in Social Groupwork Practice* has also been published as *Social Work with Groups,* Volume 6, Numbers 3/4, Fall/Winter 1983.

The Haworth Press, Inc., 28 East 22 Street, New York, NY 10010

**Library of Congress Cataloging in Publication Data**
Main entry under title:

Groupwork with women/groupwork with men.

"Has also been published as Social work with groups, volume 6, numbers 3-4, fall–winter 1983"—T.p. verso.
Includes bibliographies.
1. Social group work—Addresses, essays, lectures. 2. Women—Services for—Addresses, essays, lectures. 3. Men—Services for—Addresses, essays, lectures. 4. Leadership—Addresses, essays, lectures. I. Reed, Beth Glover. II. Garvin, Charles D.
HV45.S63 no. 3/4       361.4s           83-12745
ISBN 0-86656-258-3       [361.4]

# Groupwork with Women/ Groupwork with Men

## An Overview of Gender Issues in Social Groupwork Practice

Social Work with Groups
Volume 6, Numbers 3/4

## CONTENTS

JUDITH B. LEE, DSW, *School of Social Work, New York University, New York, New York*

BARUCH LEVINE, PhD, *Jane Addams College of Social Work, University of Illinois, and private practice, Chicago*

HENRY W. MAIER, PhD, *School of Social Work, University of Washington, Seattle*

RUTH R. MIDDLEMAN, EdD, *Raymond A. Kent School of Social Work, University of Louisville, Kentucky*

HELEN NORTHEN, PhD, *School of Social Work, University of Southern California, Los Angeles*

RUBY B. PERNELL, DSW, *School of Applied Social Sciences, Case Western Reserve University, Cleveland*

HELEN PHILLIPS, DSW, *School of Social Work, University of Pennsylvania, Philadelphia*

HERMAN RESNICK, PhD, *School of Social Work, University of Washington, Seattle*

SHELDON ROSE, PhD, *School of Social Work, University of Wisconsin, Madison*

JANICE H. SCHOPLER, MSW, *School of Social Work, University of North Carolina, Chapel Hill*

LAWRENCE SHULMAN, EdD, *School of Social Work, University of British Columbia, Vancouver, Canada*

MARY LOUISE SOMERS, DSW, *School of Social Service Administration, University of Chicago*

EMANUEL TROPP, MSSW, *School of Social Work, Virginia Commonwealth University, Richmond*

ROBERT VINTER, PhD, *School of Social Work, University of Michigan, Ann Arbor*

CELIA B. WEISMAN, DSW, *Wurzweiler School of Social Work, Yeshiva University, New York*

GERTRUDE WILSON, MA, *University of California, Berkeley*

# Groupwork with Women/ Groupwork with Men

## An Overview of Gender Issues in Social Groupwork Practice

# *EDITORIAL*

In their conception of gender issues, Charles Garvin and Beth Reed, our guest editors, adopt a forward looking view of "la difference." Avoiding polarization, there emerges from the selected papers an interactionist attention to male/female relationship, a most appropriate focus for group work service.

In the recent literature of our profession and that of all the helping professons, special attention, appropriately so, has been given to increasing our knowledge of women and women's groups. In this issue, the guest editors offer opportunity for additional understanding of men's groups and mixed groups and the gender issues that confront both men and women.

This special issue adds to the accumulation of knowledge and professional activity as men and women in our society seek out new realignments and more satisfying interrelationships.

The guest editors, Garvin and Reed, both professors at the University of Michigan School of Social Work, have had a long standing interest in this area of concern and we all benefit from their wisdom in selecting the papers and developing the issue.

*CP*
*BR*

*1*

# BASIC ISSUES

# GUEST EDITORIAL

# Gender Issues in Social Group Work: An Overview

Charles D. Garvin
Beth Glover Reed

**ABSTRACT.** This introductory essay outlines some of the reasons why a knowledge of gender is important for social group workers. We identify key concepts that are often confounded in our understanding of gender and discuss gender stereotypes and status differences between men and women and their implications for group work; we further discuss how disordered behaviors and social problems are related to these gender role stereotypes and status differences. Finally, we assert that many of the theories underlying social work practice reflect gender stereotypes, and that group work research and theory have largely ignored gender as a variable.

Each of the articles that follow in this journal address one or more ways that a knowledge of gender and its pervasive effects can inform our work in groups. The purpose of this introductory essay is to indicate why a knowledge of gender should be of central importance to everyone working with people today, and specifically, how this knowledge enters into the way we should work with groups. We will also indicate how particular articles in this journal issue seek to clarify these issues.

Charles D. Garvin, PhD, is Professor of Social Work, University of Michigan, Ann Arbor, MI 49109. Beth Glover Reed, PhD, is Associate Professor of Social Work, University of Michigan.

*5*

## GENDER AND INDIVIDUAL IDENTITY

Gender is a fundamental component of individual identity. Usually, the first words uttered about a new infant are: "It's a boy!" or "It's a girl!" In social group work, we often work with people concerned with exploring identity and self-concept issues, and many aspects of behavior that are directly or indirectly related to their gender and societal assumptions about it.

Increasingly, theorists, researchers and practitioners (e.g., Sherif, 1982; Solomon, 1982b; Shively and DeCecco, 1977) are noting that both individually and within the larger culture, we confuse separable concepts of biological gender, gender identity, gender (or sex) role behaviors, and sexual orientation or preference. This confounding leads us to mislabel many types of gender-related issues, in ways that may perpetuate unhelpful and potentially harmful gender stereotypes.

*Gender* is one's biological sex and includes chromosomal and genetic factors, sex organs and various types of secondary sex characteristics (e.g., beard, breasts). As researchers struggle to determine what human behaviors are determined by biological gender (Maccoby and Jacklin, 1974; Money, 1980), many assumed biologically based explanations of masculine and feminine behaviors have been challenged. Many are now known to vary from situation to situation, and while there clearly are some biological imperatives (e.g., menstruation), in most cases, we cannot separate biological factors from culturally determined socialization patterns. In fact, we can influence biological events via socialization and conditioning.

*Gender identity* is the inner, subjective conviction that a person is a male or female. This core belief is a major component of personality and is believed by most theorists to be immutable by the age of two or three. In contributes to the development of other affective and cognitive personality components such as body image and self-esteem.

*Gender or social sex role* is the expectations, behaviors, characteristics, norms, and role sets defined by the larger culture, the family and the self as appropriately masculine, feminine, or as unrelated to gender. Cultural beliefs and values, of course, are integrated into the behavior and thought of everyone. Gender role development begins at birth and evolves through the integration of a multitude of experiences (psychosexual, social, cognitive, moral, relationship, etc.). Changes in gender role continue through the life course, but the core of the role is usually well integrated by early adulthood, and rarely undergoes spontaneous modification (Solomon, 1982a).

Gender role assumptions and behaviors are often so completely integrated into the behavior and thought of each individual, that components of gender role expectations have become an integral part of gender identity. The actual behaviors may be relatively easy to modify, but the related beliefs and moral judgements that underlie the behaviors are much more resistant to change. Thus, attempts to change, or pressure to change the role behaviors, even if they are unsatisfying or problematic, may induce identity-related distress or even panic.

*Sexual object choice* or sexual orientation refers to the gender of the person chosen as a sexual partner. These choices can also include being autosexual or asexual. Sexual object choice is not necessarily rigidly prescribed and may change through the life course. It is frequently mistaken to be part of gender identity and gender role, an assumption that can lead to the mistaken labeling of gender identity conflicts (e.g., transexuality) or gender role issues (e.g., an assertive self-assured woman) as forms of homosexual orientations. Such mislabeling makes it difficult to identify the real source of gender-related issues, and makes work with them unnecessarily confusing and anxiety-provoking.

Remaining sensitive to the differences in these definitions and our tendency to confuse them is an integral component in the development of gender-sensitivity in our work. These issues are addressed most directly in the articles by Morson and McInnis and Gambrill and Richey, but also arise in one form or another in almost every paper in this collection.

## GENDER ROLE STEREOTYPES
## AND STATUS DIFFERENCES

### Cultural Stereotypes about Appropriate Masculine and Feminine Role Behaviors

Many researchers have demonstrated the presence of widely shared conceptions of what this culture defines as appropriate masculine and feminine characteristics and behaviors (e.g., females are affectively and socioemotionally oriented; males are instrumentally and competitively oriented). Until fairly recently, masculinity and femininity were defined as bipolar concepts, i.e., as opposites. In fact, most people still talk about the "opposite sex." Boys and girls are socialized to behave in ways consistent with these stereotypes.

The work of Bem (1974), Kaplan and Bean (1976), and others on androgeny challenges this bipolar conceptualization of gender roles. The concept is derived from the Greek ando (male) and gyn (female) to suggest a flexible integration in a single person, of characteristics usually associated with women or men, a person who has moved beyond scientific and cultural stereotypes for her or his gender. While some men and women perceive themselves and behave in accordance with traditional sex-role stereotypes, others are able to use the positive attributes associated with both masculine and feminine stereotypes. Thus, to increase many clients' coping and adaptive capacities, workers must help them to explore their gender socialization and the skills and orientations that were enhanced or inhibited by this socialization.

One of the consequences of having different views of what is appropriate behavior for each gender is that people then use different standards of judgement when they evaluate identical behaviors in women compared to men. Gambrill and Richey describe some of the ways that these different standards of judgement can influence social skills training—in assessment, identification of target behaviors, selecting intervention strategies and evaluating results.

Most of the articles in this issue address the consequences of polarized gender socialization, and many describe ways that people can explore its consequences and develop alternatives for themselves. Stein, Kaufman and Timmers, Currie, and Buckley et al. discuss some of the ways these issues can be explored in all-male groups while Gottlieb et al., Adolph, Haussmann and Halseth, Hagen and Hartman explore the issues as they arise in all-female groups as women work on relationship and autonomy issues and becoming more assertive. Reed and Bernardez address some of the ways that our gender role stereotypes and socialization influence the ways we react to women leaders in groups.

## Status Differences between Women and Men

A sex role perspective alone emphasizes the complementarity of male and female roles, but ignores the process of power and prestige ordering that occurs when men and women interact. There is considerable evidence that women's and men's roles are not valued equally by society, that men's contributions are more valued than women's not only monetarily, but also in terms of status and prestige, and that these status differences influence male and female behaviors in group settings (Lockheed & Hall, 1976; Meeker & Weitzel-O'Neill, 1977). Several of the articles in this journal review this literature, notably Martin and Shanahan, Gambrill and Richey, and Reed. People who have more status display both verbal and non-verbal behaviors that indicate more dominance and power (they talk more often, address the entire group, are less personal); those with lower status are more deferent verbally and non-verbally. Those socialized for higher status positions often resist accepting this view of themselves and its possible consequences, and may fear that role change will lead to a loss of some advantages associated with the higher status. Those with lower status are likely to have incorporated some of the consequences of this position into their self-image and worldview. Self-esteem is often low, they may feel very isolated, and are more likely to blame themselves for their circumstances.

These behaviors and self-perceptions are also consistent with gender socialization practices and stereotypes, although Kanter (1977a, 1977b, 1977c) has demonstrated that even men, when placed in positions of low status without access to advancement and sources of power and influence, behave in ways defined as stereotypically feminine. Thus, status-related behaviors and self-perceptions do not just arise from socialization but are also related to environmental factors and will change if the environment changes or if status variables (e.g., legitimization) are adjusted. Education about these relationships and the multiple origins of many gender-related perceptions and behaviors will be very important components of group work with both women and men.

Status differences between women and men must be considered in planning group composition and in working with both men and women in the same group (noted especially by Martin & Shanahan). They also influence what occurs in all-men and all-women groups. Nine of the articles in this collection discuss work primarily in single gender groups and all of them discuss different aspects of status-related dynamics and how they can be addressed. Reed and Bernardez present some of the ways that status and socialization interact to generate different reactions to women group leaders, and

Gambrill and Richey describe status as a key characteristic to consider in social skills training groups.

## GENDER-LINKED DISORDERS AND SOCIAL PROBLEMS

Behavioral disorders that occur most frequently in each gender are highly related to gender roles and socialization (e.g., Lewis, 1976; Gomberg & Franks, 1979). Those most common in women usually have major affective components (e.g., depression, anxiety, cyclic mood disorders, extreme dependency), or body-image distortions (e.g., anorexia). Those for men more often have major cognitive components (thought disorders, obsessive compulsive patterns) or involve taking action rather than facing problems (sexual disorders, alcoholism, violence). These patterns suggest the extremes of gender stereotyping, almost as if masculine and feminine socialization has been *too* successful. The types of problems that bring members of each gender to social workers are also often directly related to gender-linked circumstances—low income and child care responsibilities, gynecological problems, and as victims of violence for women; for men, vocational, criminal, or violence related problems, or particular health problems (e.g., heart).

Knowledge about gender differences, socialization, societal contributions to male and female-linked behaviors, and knowledge about how to change these assumptions and behaviors will be crucial in working with many of these disorders more effectively. Stein discusses some of these problems for men; Haussman and Halseth describe a group for depressed rural women while Adolph reports on use of feminist and consciousness-raising group techniques with women in a psychiatric day hospital. A cluster of articles by Hartman, Currie, and Buckley et al. describe several modes of working with domestic violence—a group of women who have been battered and groups for men who have battered.

## CHANGING GENDER ROLES

Our society is one of rapid changes and these have had profound consequences for sex roles. For women, many of these changes are due to the fact that they are "living longer, marrying later, and less often, remarrying less frequently, having and expecting to have fewer children, and more often than previously, planning to have no children" (Lipman-Blumen, 1976). This has led to an increase in women living alone as well as heading families as single parents.

While male domination of higher education, particularly at a graduate level, continues, the situation in the work force has been changing. The proportion of women employed continues to grow and a majority of wives are now employed. While women with young children are less likely to work than those without, even this category of women workers has been increasing. The type of employment secured by women has also been changing so that, while women are still more likely to be in certain blue and pink collar occupations as well as "traditional" fields such as teaching, nursing, and secretarial work, their entry into all other fields is on the increase. Nevertheless, they are severely underrepresented in most high status professions and occupations and they are not likely to be paid as adequately as men for the same work.

The above demographic changes have been associated with and are often fueled by other social changes including the development of the women's movement, changed roles for men and women in the family, and the emergence of new family forms altogether. The major concerns of the women's movement have been removing sex stereotyping of jobs, creating job opportunities for women, fighting unequal pay for women, encouraging work outside the home, eliminating sexism in all spheres of life activity, and protecting women against violence.

A men's movement has also been emerging, undoubtedly, in part, as a consequence of the women's movement. Seven annual conferences on "Men and Masculinity" have been held and a national men's organization is being organized. Men's and women's consciousness raising activities have been initiated to help men and women cope with the way sexism affects them. Men's activities seek to help them to uncover and cope with their propensity to use violence and competition, as well as to suppress their emotions as well as their desires to develop close and supportive relationships with other men.

All of these issues are associated with changes in family life. These include a movement toward sharing roles that were originally sexually stereotyped including household chores, child care, child socialization, and the production of income (Nye, 1976). These changes, however, have usually not produced a totally egalitarian family and, in fact, may have created an increase in tensions in the family as current demands and previous socialization confront each other.

## GENDER BIASES IN PRACTICE

Our work with parents, teachers, family members, etc. will be influenced by how we have been taught, and reinforced or punished for, sex role behaviors. For example, do we promote parents' awareness of whether their expectations of their children perpetuate sex role stereotypes? Of whether daughters are punished for assertiveness and sons for signs of passivity or weakness?

One set of contemporary practice ideas stem from an understanding of the family as a system. We see this as a progressive development in the growth of our knowledge base, particularly in the way such knowledge helps us to understand the social bases of behavior. We find it strange, nevertheless, that so little of the practice literature on family therapy stresses the effect of gender issues on the problems presented by families. Family therapy writings are replete with discussions of many types of conflicts between spouses yet the relevance to this of how men and women are socialized to deal with power issues is usually ignored. Parent-child conflicts are another major category of problems considered in the family therapy literature yet how such conflicts relate to sex role socialization conflicts for both parent and child is similarly not injected into the analysis.

An understanding of gender issues can lead to a useful reexamination of family dynamics. In a family, for example, with a young adolescent daughter who was labeled anorexic, the worker failed to see that the expectations of this youngster, as well as her sisters, were linked to an overemphasis on physical appearance and that these expectations did not extend to the brothers. Similarly, the worker was able to see that the mother "subtly" manipulated her husband and children in ways that perpetuated family problems, but did not see that the entire family's attitude toward female assertiveness made it difficult for the mother to express her wishes directly.

Gender issues related to the family are often reflected in groups because of their potential to recreate family dynamics. How men and women use power and assume roles in the family, and participate in family decision making are often transferred to the group situation. The reasons for joining the group may even be explicitly to resolve family situations. This makes it important for workers and members to explore parallels between the family and group so that members may obtain satisfactory resolution of gender issues in both places.

In many settings in which social workers have central responsibility for socialization experiences (such as in child welfare programs), the group is the media for much of this work. Workers hold "cottage" meetings in child welfare institutions and groups are similarly used in rehabilitation, correctional, and school settings. Workers must have a full understanding of contemporary issues in sex role socialization in order to operate non-sexist programs in these circumstances. We find, too often, that workers either perpetuate traditional roles or interpret gender issues psychologically rather than see the contribution of social forces to sex role socialization.

Human services often have direct responsibility for the socialization of individuals. Foster care, institutional, and peer group programs conducted by social workers directly involve sex role socialization. Do the workers in these endeavors avoid gender stereotypes, help consumers of services to make choices related to gender, and provide a range of sex role models?

Another gender issue in human services is how well the workers understand the contribution of gender factors to the kinds of problems and their solutions brought by clients. Is male violence, for example, understood as men carrying to an extreme violent ways of behaving that are impressed upon the minds of most males in our society? Are depressed women understood as often reaping the consequences of their deprivation of power and their response to this? Is the larger percentage of women seeking mental health services correctly understood not as an intrinsic weakness in women or their wish to depend upon others but rather as a sign of the limited ways women have available to them to influence their environments?

Another issue for social workers is to examine critically the theories they draw upon for their appropriateness for both men and women, and we offer a few examples. Psychoanalytic theory has heavily influenced social work practice yet social scientists with a feminist perspective have levelled criticisms at Freud's ideas about gender (Frieze et al., 1978). Currently, practitioners and researchers are reexamining psychoanalytic and other personality theories incorporating perspectives and knowledge gained from the new scholarship on women and men. This work is very exciting, and sometimes controversial, but is likely to transform many basic assumptions about gender identity and role development with many implications for social group work and other forms of practice (e.g., Chodorow, 1974, 1978; Miller, 1976; Wyckoff, 1977; Solomon & Levy, 1982; Brodsky & Hare-Mustin, 1980; Rawlings & Carter, 1977).

Gender issues are also embedded in the profession and in the service delivery system. We believe, along with Kadushin, that there are practice consequences of the large proportion of social workers in direct practice who are women compared to the proportion of social work administrators who are men (Kadushin, 1976). This condition should be considered along with the fact that many other professions with whom social workers interact, such as physicians, are predominantly male.

We discussed earlier the problem of theories that perpetuate sexist ideas. We offered as examples psychoanalytic and family therapies as both of these have an impact on all interpersonal helping. There are also ideas that are specifically relevant to group work practice that may be used in sexist ways. Any theory, for example, that deals with group composition, leadership, cohesiveness, and structure should be examined for failures to distinguish between the responses of men and women. Women and men are likely to use power and handle opportunities for intimacy differently from each other. Similarly, subgroups in men's groups are more likely to form around patterns of competitiveness than in women's groups where patterns of similarity of interest and attitude are important determinants of structure. These are just a few of the many pieces of information that should be incorporated in our understanding of small group processes so that the worker can help members to develop satisfying sex role identities for themselves.

## Lack of Knowledge about Impact of Gender on Group Dynamics

Until recently, there was no attention to gender in groups except to document stereotypically masculine and feminine behaviors in men and women respectively and attribute them to biological factors or socialization practices. As noted earlier, more recently these findings have been reinterpreted using theories about diffuse status states (see Martin & Shanahan this volume for a summary) and an examination of the gender composition within the group.

Further attention to gender composition and its effects is yielding important information about all-male and all-female groups (see Stein, Kaufman & Timmers, Gottleib et al., and Hagen) and how they can be used effectively. Study of mixed groups suggests that they have different effects on men and women, and that many of their effects for women act to restrict their role options and relegate them to less powerful positions within the group. Some ways to deal with these dynamics are presented in the Martin and Shanahan, Gambrill and Richey, and Reed and Bernardez articles.

The effects of leader gender have also been little studied. Almost the entire theory and research on group development and other group characteristics has been conducted on groups with men leaders (and usually with men members). If a women leader was included, this is often not noted, and data from women-led groups was not examined separately. As a result, we know very little about the effects of female leadership on member perceptions, behaviors, or on group development, structure, and so forth. What is known is reviewed by Reed and Bernardez in this volume with an emphasis on its implications for leaders and members.

## FUTURE TASKS

We believe that the authors in this volume have done an excellent job of beginning the presentation of important gender issues that should inform all of social group work practice. Nevertheless, we are acutely aware of many issues that have not yet been adequately researched or explored thus far, and that should be the next items on this "agenda." Among these are:

1. There are many differences in gender socialization and role definitions among various ethnic groups. While black or Hispanic or Native American women and men, to mention a few groups, are exposed to the sex role stereotypes and status differences that affect us all, they also have unique traditions and histories. There is an emerging literature on this topic that should be expanded, in its own right, as well as used to generate relevant ideas for group experiences useful for women and men that are also ethnically sensitive. We also know very little as yet about the interaction among different leader status characteristics—e.g., gender, ethnicity, age. We

have addressed some of the consequences of having a woman leader in a small group, but what if she is also black?

2. Since many groups conducted by social group workers involve children and youth, we must clarify how an understanding of gender differences at particular ages, gender socialization, and gender-related group dynamics can be applied in groups with children whose gender-role behaviors, self concepts, and sexual identities are still developing.

3. We must continue to develop our understanding of how (so-called) mental illness is maintained by gender issues in our society. All forms of group work in mental health settings should be informed by this knowledge.

4. All models and techniques of group work have gender implications and are not gender "neutral." Gambrill and Richey, for example, identify some of the gender issues in social skills training in this volume. The same kind of analysis must be conducted for all of the approaches we use as social group workers.

5. While the article by Morson and McInnis begins the task of separating sexual preference issues from those of gender, gender identity, and gender roles, much more must be done to overcome the many stereotypes we hold regarding the labeling of gay men and lesbians and continue to explore the gender issues involved in exploring sexual identity. Our societal confounding of the various aspects of sexual identity virtually forces gay men and lesbians to examine their values and assumptions about gender, gender identity, and gender role behaviors in order to integrate sexual orientation issues with other aspects of gender and sexual identities and behaviors. Thus, group work with gay men and lesbians is likely to provide valuable insights and information about how these components can be "unconfounded" whatever one's sexual orientation.

6. Finally, much more research must be conducted on the various ways that gender can affect groups of different sizes, composition and goals, and, as our knowledge about the effects of gender on social group work practice expands, as it should, the information must be organized to provide a coherent set of guidelines and suggestions for practitioners. This volume only scratches the surface given our time and space limitations. Many interesting practice illustrations could already be in-

cluded here, like the very interesting work by Bernardez and
Stein (1979) who have experimented with alternately using
single gender and mixed groups and also switching male and
female leaders to provide members with comparative experiences of their own reactions and behaviors to both leader
gender and group composition. More such experimentation
and research need to be developed.

## REFERENCES

Bem, S. L. The measurement of psychological Androgyny. *Journal of Consulting and Clinical Psychology*, 1974, *42*, 155-162.
_____. Sex-role adaptability: One consequence of psychological androgyny. *Journal of
Personality and Social Psychology*, 1975, *31*, 634-643.
Bernardez, T. and Stein, T. S. Separating the sexes in group therapy: An experiment with
men's and women's groups. *International Journal of Group Psychotherapy, 29*, 1979,
493-502.
Brodsky, A. and Hare-Mustin, R., (eds). *Women and psychotherapy: An assessment of re-
search and practice.* New York: Guilford Press, 1980.
Chodorow, N. Family structure and feminine personality. In M. R. Rosaldo and L. Lam-
phere, eds., *Women, culture and society.* Stanford, CA: Stanford University Press, 1974.
Chodorow, N. *The reproduction of mothering.* Berkeley, CA: University of California
Press, 1978.
Frieze, I. H., et al. *Women and sex roles.* New York: W. W. Norton, 1978.
Gomberg, E. S. and Franks, V. *Gender and disordered behavior: Sex differences in psycho-
pathology.* New York: Brunner/Mazel, Inc., 1979.
Kadushin, A. Men in a women's profession. *Social Work*, 1976, *21* (November).
Kanter, R. M. Men and women of the corporation. New York: Basic Books, 1977(a).
Kanter, R. M. Some effects of proportions in group life: Skewed sex ratios and responses
to token women. *American Journal of Sociology*, 1977(b), *82*, 965-990.
Kanter, R. M. Women in organizations: Sex roles, group dynamics, and change strategies.
In A. Sargent, ed. *Beyond sex roles.* St. Paul, MN: West Publishing Co., 1977(c).
Kaplan, A. G. and Bean, J. B., eds. *Beyond sex role stereotypes: Readings toward a psy-
chology of androgyny.* Boston: Little, Brown, and Co., 1976.
Lewis, G. L. Changes in women's role participation. In I. B. Frieze, et al. *Women and
sex roles.* New York: W. W. Norton, 1978, 137-156.
Lewis, H. B. *Psychic war in men and women.* New York: New York University Press, 1976.
Lipman-Blumen, J. The implications of changing sex roles for family structure. In C. Mun-
son, ed. *Social work with families.* New York: Free Press, 1980, 99-118.
Lockheed, M. E. and Hall, K. P. Conceptualizing sex as a status characteristic: Applica-
tions to leadership training strategies. *Journal of Social Issues*, 1976, *32*, 111-124.
Maccoby, E. E. and Jacklin, C. N. *The psychology of sex differences.* Stanford, CA: Stan-
ford University Press, 1974.
Meeker, B. F. and Weitzel-O'Neill, P. A. Sex roles and interpersonal behavior in task
oriented groups. *American Sociological Review*, 1977, *42*, 91-105.
Miller, J. B. *Toward a new psychology of women.* Boston: Beacon Press, 1976.
Money, J. *Love and love sickness: The science of sex gender difference, and pair bonding.*
Baltimore: Johns Hopkins University Press, 1980.
Nye, F. I. *Role structure and analysis of the family.* Beverly Hills, CA: Sage Publications,
1976.

Rawlings, E. and Carter, D., eds. *Psychotherapy for women: Treatment towards equality.* Springfield, IL: Charles C Thomas, 1977.

Sherif, C. W. Needed concepts in the study of gender identity. *Psychology of Women Quarterly,* 1982, *6,* 375-398.

Shively, M. G. and DeCecco, J. P. Components of sexual identity. *Journal of Homosexuality,* 1977, *3*(1), 41-48.

Solomon, K. Individual psychotherapy and the changing roles of men: Dimensions of gender role psychotherapy. In K. Solomon and N. B. Levy, eds. *Men in transition: Changing male roles, theory, and therapy.* New York: Plenum Press, 1982(a).

Solomon, K. Counseling the drug dependent women: Special issues for men. In B. G. Reed, G. M. Beschner, and J. Mondanaro. *Treatment services for drug dependent women,* Vol. II. Rockville, MD: National Institute on Drug Abuse, DHHS Pub No (ADM) 82-1219. 1982, 572-612.

Solomon, K. and Levy, N. B., eds. *Men in transition: Changing male roles, theory, and therapy.* New York: Plenum Press, 1982.

Wyckoff, H. *Solving women's problems.* New York: Grove Press, 1977.

# Transcending the Effects
# of Sex Composition in Small Groups

Patricia Yancey Martin
Kristin A. Shanahan

**ABSTRACT.** A review of recent literature (1976 to 1982) on the topic of sex composition of small groups summarizes three theoretical explanations for male-female differences in same and mixed sex groups (including sex role differentiation; status characteristics/expectation states theory; and Kanter's structural/numerical proportions model); and five categories of empirical findings (including non-verbal effects; verbal interaction frequency and content; negative assessments of influential females; negative consequences of "token" or "solo" status for females; and contradictions in findings regarding all-female groups). Interventions for transcending group sex composition effects are identified for both women and men in mixed and same sex groups. Conclusions call for additional research, utilizing methods with high internal and external validity, on the effects of sex composition in treatment and "real-world" work groups.

The literature on gender, gender composition of groups, and small group structure and process leaves little doubt that the "sex composition" of small groups entails dramatic implications for group functioning and outcomes. Understanding the effects of sex composition is important for several reasons. First, almost no study which investigates the effects of group sex composition (to be defined shortly) finds it unimportant—either alone or in combination with other variables, whether these are perceptual (e.g., attitudes), behavioral (e.g., statements made, actions taken, or goals accomplished), or both.

Patricia Yancey Martin is a Professor of Social Work and Sociology at The Florida State University in Tallahassee, FL 32306. Kristin A. Shanahan is a social work graduate student at The Florida State University, Tallahassee. Requests for reprints should be sent to Patricia Martin, School of Social Work, The Florida State University, Tallahassee, FL 32306.

Second, considerable evidence indicates that the effects of sex composition are so pervasive and subtle they are activated merely by visual perception—that is, independently of verbal exchanges or other forms of social interaction. Simply the presence in one physical setting of a particular gender mix or configuration has been observed to affect subjects' attitudes towards feminism (Shomer & Centers, 1970) ratings of others' "emotional appeal" or attractiveness (Berman, O'Nan, & Floyd, 1981), and assessment of females' work orientations and leadership potential (Frank & Katcher, 1977).

Third, and perhaps most importantly, a cumulating body of evidence suggests that interventions on the part of a group leader or experimenter can successfully counteract many otherwise undesirable effects of a group's given gender configuration (see, for example, Lockheed & Hall, 1976; Piliavin & Martin, 1978; Fennell, Barchas, Cohen, McMahon, & Hildebrand, 1978; Ridgeway, 1982).

A primary aim of this article is to enhance awareness of tactics or techniques which can be used to "neutralize" undesirable effects of group sex composition. Since some research suggests that females' behaviors and attitudes are affected more strongly than males' by contextual influences such as group sex composition (see, for example, Piliavin & Martin, 1978; Israeli, 1983), particular attention is paid to the effects of group sex composition on females.

This review focuses primarily on theoretical and empirical work published between 1976 and 1982 which deals with the effects of sex composition in small (3 to 10 members, typically) face-to-face groups. Research on dyads is excluded. The concept of *group sex composition* refers to the "proportional mix" of group members in relation to sex. Group sex composition can take a variety of forms. A *uniform group* is either 100 percent male or 100 percent female (Kanter, 1977a, 1977b). Groups with both male and female members are called mixed groups. Following Kanter (1977a, 1977b), mixed groups can be of three general types: (1) *skewed* with a mix which entails only one or very few of one category (e.g., 15 percent female; 85 percent male); (2) *tilted* with a mix which is somewhat less imbalanced than in a skewed group (e.g., 25 percent female, 75 percent male); and (3) *balanced* which contains nearly equal proportions of males and females (e.g., 40 to 60 percent of each). A single member of one gender in an otherwise opposite sex (skewed) group is referred to in the literature as a "solo" (Wolman

& Frank, 1975) or "token" (Kanter, 1977a, 1977b) member. Use of the term solo or token is usually reserved, however, for the lower-status (e.g., female, black) single member in an otherwise higher-status (e.g., male, white) group (see Kanter, 1977a).

In the review, we summarize: (1) the primary theoretical perspectives from the literature on male-female differences in same sex and mixed sex groups; and (3) some of the more consistently observed empirical results of group sex composition for both males and females. Additionally, an overview of strategies is presented for transcending the effects of gender in groups and suggestions are offered for future research regarding the consequences of sex composition in both discussion/treatment and task/work types of groups.

## OVERVIEW OF THE LITERATURE

In the empirical articles reviewed, four distinctive "types of groups" are found. These are: (1) experimental task groups (i.e., groups with a "group-level" objective, where participants are "evaluated" regarding progress towards the objective; Shomer & Centers, 1970; Eskilson & Wiley, 1976; Fennell, Barchas, Cohen, McMahon, & Hildebrand, 1978; Patterson & Shaeffer, 1977; Ridgeway & Jacobson, 1977; Berman, O'Nan, & Floyd, 1981; Bradley, 1980; and Ridgeway, 1982); (2) actual work groups (Wolman & Frank, 1975; Frank & Katcher, 1977; Kanter, 1977a, 1977b; Izraeli, 1983; and Note 1; and South, Bonjean, Markham, & Corder, 1982 and Note 2); (2) experimental discussion groups (subjects randomly assigned and directed to interact verbally but without collective "evaluation" regarding progress towards group goals; Aires, 1976; Piliavin & Martin, 1978); and (3) growth/therapy groups (groups which met over time with specific growth or therapeutic goals for individual participants; Carlock & Martin, 1977; Green, Morrison, & Tischler, 1980; Thune, Manderscheid, & Silbergeld, 1980). Two articles failed to examine "small groups" per se but are nevertheless included due to their examination of sex composition effects of the broader social context (Szafran, Note 4; Spangler, Gordon, & Pipkin, 1978). It should be noted that over two-thirds of the empirical works reviewed were based either on experimental task or "real-world" work groups. Present results are necessarily, therefore, more applicable to task/work than to growth/ therapeutic group contexts.

*Theoretical Models.* Until recently, the primary theoretical explanation for differences in women's and men's behavior in groups rested on a "sex roles differentiation" model (for accounts of this model, see Lockheed & Hall, 1976; Fennell et al., 1978; Meeker & Weitzer-O'Neill, 1977; Thune et al., 1980). This model focuses attention on the *personal attributes* of participants in relation to childhood (and later) socialization into the socio-cultural roles of "male" and "female." For example, the sex role differentiation model suggests that males talk, direct, and dominate more than females in groups *because* they have been socialized to be "task/ instrumental" specialists whereas females talk, direct, and dominate less because they have been socialized to be "socio-emotional/expressive" specialists. Such a "division of labor" can be expected because it is consistent with the division of labor in the home where the male/husband/father is the "task" leader and the female/wife/mother is the "socio-emotional" leader. Although recent analyses challenge this view (see Meeker & Weitzel-O'Neill, 1977), sociologists in the 1950s contended that such a division of labor between the sexes was natural, inevitable, and "functional" for the preservation of the family (see, for example, Bales & Slater, 1955). The sex role differentiation explanation is now viewed by many as both simplistic and pessimistic—simplistic because it tells only part of the story and pessimistic because it implies that little can be done to modify differential male-female interaction patterns in group contexts.

Since the mid-seventies, the theoretical model most widely used to account for male/female differences in groups is a "status characteristics/expectation states" model (see Berger, Cohen, & Zelditch, 1972; Berger, Fisek, Norman, & Zelditch, 1977; Meeker & Weitzel-O'Neill, 1977; Webster & Driskell, 1978). This model directs attention to *status and situational rather than personal* factors to account for male-female differences. Gender is viewed as a *diffuse,* as opposed to specific, *status characteristic* which is "defined" in the broader society (external to the group) and which entails "expectations" (from both self and others) for normatively appropriate behaviors in social contexts. The term diffuse means that expectations for behavior associated with gender status (i.e., male or female) are "known" by most societal members and, lacking evidence to the contrary, are assumed to be widely applicable. They are, therefore, "brought into" most social situations.

If males are viewed normatively as more appropriate "task

leaders'' than females are—and, as ample evidence suggests, this is the case in most developed societies (Martin, Harrison, & DiNitto, 1982; Stacey, Note 3)—males will therefore *act* this way, more so than females, *unless* interventions are instituted to neutralize the expectations which foster such behaviors. In this model, ''males act like males'' and ''females act like females'' in small groups because: (a) their gender is obvious to all; (b) the normative expectations associated with their gender are well known to all and assumed to be widely applicable; and (c) compliance with expectations associated with one's gender status is rewarded and non-compliance, negatively sanctioned. This perspective allows for a conceptual ''separation'' of an individual from his/her behavior and suggests that a person may wish to, and know how to, behave differently from the norms associated with his/her gender status. The status characteristics/expectations states model suggests, therefore, that social *norms* associated with gender status stimulate certain expectations which in turn foster certain behaviors. In contrast to the sex role differentiation model, this model is optimistic because it suggests that alteration of the normative structure of a social situation can also alter members' expectations and associated behaviors.

Kanter (1977a, 1977b) has recently articulated a ''structural/numerical proportions'' model which explicates the relationship between *the relative proportion of males and females* in a group and the perceptions and experiences of group members. She argues that groups composed mostly of majority/male members and only one or a few minority/female members influence the male members to experience ''perceptual distortions'' regarding the ''token'' female's characteristics and actions. As a result, behaviors of the female are seen as ''representative of all women'' rather than those of an individual person. Stemming from the males' perceptual distortions, female members are subjected to heightened visibility, performance pressures, and role entrapment (see Kanter, 1977a).

Kanter's recommended solution for preventing such ''perceptual distortions'' and their attendant dynamics is to ''equalize'' small groups on the proportional representation of male and female members. When this occurs, she claims that each member is more likely to be viewed as an individual and that stereotype-related norms are less likely to be invoked. Recent empirical work by Spangler, Gordon, and Pipkin (1978) and Izraeli (1983; Note 1) lend support to Kanter's model, particularly for females in mixed groups. (Also, see South et al., 1982 and Note 2, who support

Kanter's claims that proportional representation is important and that female tokens are negatively treated. Their work does not fully support, however, her claimed positive effects for females of a "balanced" gender ratio in work groups.)

*Empirical Findings.* Few empirical investigations of group sex composition study the same dependent variables. The following summary is therefore selective and attempts to reflect the range and diversity, rather than depth, of reported findings.

1. *Even without interpersonal interaction (e.g., verbal exchanges), females are negatively "evaluated" in all-male groups and in groups in which they are tokens* (Frank & Katcher, 1977; Berman, O'Nan, & Floyd, 1981; Shomer & Centers, 1970). Research of this type lends support to status characteristics/expectation states theory in its claim that evaluations based on gender enter group contexts as a result of generalized expectations and "values" learned in the external society.

2. *The quantity and content of verbal interaction in groups varies by group sex composition and by gender of participant.* Several studies report that women talk (initiate interaction) less and are talked to less in mixed groups than in all-female groups (Aries, 1976; Carlock & Martin, 1977; Piliavin & Martin, 1978). Aries (1976) found that males in all-male groups tend to concentrate on competition and status topics whereas females in all-female groups focus on personal, home, and family topics. In mixed groups, male comments changed in the direction of the females; males talked more about themselves and their feelings and exhibited a more personal orientation. Females in mixed groups talked less about their personal views but did not increase their other types of comments. Similar to Aries, Piliavin and Martin (1978) report changes in content of interaction from same sex to mixed sex groups. Whereas males emitted similar proportions of "instrumental/task" and "socio-emotional/expressive" comments in mixed as in all-male groups (about 72% to 20%), they showed less disagreement and conflict in mixed groups. Females, on the other hand, increased slightly their instrumental (in contrast to expressive) comments in mixed groups (over all-female) and showed somewhat more disagreement. Piliavin and Martin (1978) conclude that both males and females interact verbally in less "sex role stereotyped" ways in positive, task-related verbal statements to "leader-like" behavior, Eskilson and Wiley (1976) found both males and females to exhibit the greatest quantity of "leader-like" statements in same sex groups. Females

acted "least leader-like" when leading two males (in three-person groups); males acted least leader-like when their followers were one male and one female.

3. *Females are perceived of less positively than males; even when equally "influential."* Bradley (1980) and Ridgeway (1982) found that female confederates (persons trained to participate in experiments) in otherwise all-male groups were not well liked (based on the males' subjective assessments) even though they were highly "influential" in relation to group decision-making. Izraeli (1983) found, in Israeli union executive committees, that regardless of group sex composition, males were much more likely than females to view men as "better leaders" than women. Female members, on the other hand, were more influenced in their views of leadership ability by their committee's sex composition: women in balanced groups (close to a 50/50 male/female membership) *viewed women as slightly better leaders than men* whereas women in skewed groups (15% or fewer women and 85% of more men) saw men as better leaders than women. Highly influential females in all-female groups were found by Ridgeway (1982) to be less well-liked than those whose influence was lower.

4. *"Solo" or "token" females in otherwise male groups tend to fare poorly.* Wolman and Frank (1975) report that four of six "solo" women in professional peer groups felt they were "pushed into deviant roles" by their male peers. Frank and Katcher (1977) found that in small work groups, solo females were perceived by male group members as "low in work orientation" even before interpersonal exchanges occurred. This was not the case, however, when more than one woman was present. Kanter (1977a, 1977b) reports that token females are placed under unusual pressures—leading to negative outcomes—in otherwise all-male groups. Recent research by South et al. (1982; Note 2) and Izraeli (1973; Note 1) confirms this view. Research by Bradley (1980) confirms the negative assessments received by token females in otherwise male groups if no "interventions" are instituted. Confederate females trained to be "competent" at the group's task were, however, equally as successful and well-liked as "competent" males. Bradley's findings lend support to "expectation states" theory by demonstrating the ability of interventions to overcome the status disadvantage (Ridgeway, 1982) associated with female gender in mixed sex groups (also, see Bartol, 1975).

5. *Women in all-female groups: inconsistent findings.* Research

on all-female groups reveals numerous contradictions. Female-only growth or discussion groups are generally observed to be "superior" to mixed groups (for female participants). Aries (1976) found that females in all-female groups looked forward to the next meeting of their group more so than females in mixed groups (whereas males in mixed groups looked forward more than males in all-male groups did). Carlock and Martin (1977) report females in an all-female group experienced greater (positive) "objective" growth than those in a mixed group but subjectively evaluated the experience as less "exciting" and enjoyable. Females in the mixed group expressed preferences, however, for an all-female group in the future.

In task groups, Ridgeway and Jacobson (1977) report that female members perceived male confederates as "more influential" than female confederates, even though they exhibited similar behaviors. Females also gave higher "rewards" (through cash payments at the end of the game) to males than to females. Ridgeway (1982) examined the influence attempts of female confederates in all-female groups in relation to "motivation" (group vs. self) exhibited by the confederate. Contrary to her hypothesis, "self oriented" female confederates in all-female groups were much more influential than those who showed a "group orientation." (The opposite was observed for female confederates in otherwise male groups.) Ridgeway (1982, pp. 82-83) concludes that "Coming from another female, blatantly self-interested claims seemed to be perceived by females as a power play which, while resented, was largely successful." This conclusion is supported by Baker (1982) who found women in an all-female radical social movement organization to be ambivalent towards "influence" attempts and authority in their ranks.

For both males and females, Ridgeway (1982) found "likeability" to vary with motivation. Group-motivated confederates were much better liked that self-motivated confederates. This posed an anomaly in all-female groups since "group oriented" confederates were well liked but ignored (in regards to influence on the group) whereas "self-oriented" confederates were disliked but influential. Ridgeway (1982, p. 85) concludes that "These results show the complexity of the influence process in a group composed entirely of members with the low state of a diffuse status characteristic like sex." Eskilson and Wiley (1976) found that all-female (three-person) task groups with a female leader were the *least effective* (effective defined as the shortest time for completion of the group assigned task) of any group type. (All-male groups with a male leader were the most effective.) This is interesting in light of their concurrent finding that female leaders in all-female groups made a high proportion of "leader-like" verbal statements, suggesting that they attempted—unsuccessfully—to lead. Eskilson and Wiley (1976) conclude, consistent with Ridgeway (1982), that females' discomfort in assuming leadership roles and their emphasis on cooperation may hamper the success of all-female task groups in completing task assignments (also see Meeker & Weitzel-O'Neill, 1977; Piliavin & Martin, 1978; Thune, et al., 1980).

In contrast to the foregoing, recent work by Fennell et al. (1978) finds all-female groups to outperform (make "superior gain scores" to) all-male groups on a task which required explicit cooperation and a unanimous group decision. This suggests that the *type of task* a group is assigned may interact with the group's sex composition to influence group outcomes. If this is true, much of the extant research on sex composition of task groups may have to be discounted because assigned tasks are typically "numerical" or "mechanical" in nature and tasks of this type are normatively associated with the male, rather than the female, gender. Such a consideration may account for Eskilson and Wiley's (1976, p. 192) conclusion that ". . . task completion did not appear salient to groups of three females."

## TRANSCENDING GROUP SEX COMPOSITION: SUGGESTIONS FOR INTERVENTION

Interventions for group leaders interested in transcending undesirable effects of a given sex composition are summarized briefly in four categories: women in mixed groups; women in all-female groups; men in mixed groups; and men in all-male groups.

*Women in Mixed Groups.* Four avenues of intervention are suggested in the literature for transcending "status disadvantages" faced by women in mixed groups. These include (1) legitimation; (2) competency; (3) motivation; and (4) numerical proportions.

The most widely heralded intervention is that of *legitimation* which refers primarily to actions by those in authority to affirm the right of a female to assume influence, leadership, or other task-related roles (Fennell et al., 1978; Lockheed & Hall, 1976; Meeker

& Weitzel-O'Neill, 1977; Piliavin & Martin 1978). Fennell et al. (1978) suggest that women's presumed lesser success at exercising authority at work is often a result of the failure of higher-ups to support a woman's as opposed to a man's authority (also see Kanter, 1977b; Wiley & Eskilson, 1982). Piliavin and Martin (1978) found that simple encouragement of a female to talk in a mixed group increased not only her frequency of speaking but also her proportion of task-related comments. Eskilson and Wiley (1976) found female leaders who believed their leadership resulted from their own achievement—as opposed to chance—to behave in more "leader-like" ways than other females. Izraeli (1983; Note 1) found females who were elected as chairpersons of their union committees to perceive themselves as equally influential as elected male chairpersons, suggesting that "legitimacy of position" overcame otherwise potentially debilitating gender-specific expectations (e.g., "men are better leaders than women").

A second intervention entails demonstration by females of *competence* relevant to the group's assigned task(s). Recent research by Bradley (1980) found competent females in otherwise male task groups to receive high rewards from male peers. Competent females were rewarded, in fact, more than competent males! (Incompetent females were, on the other hand, assessed more negatively than incompetent males.) Bradley suggests that the "surprise element" of a solo female showing expertise in the group's assigned task area may have positively affected male colleagues' evaluation of her contributions.

A third intervention for women in mixed groups involves the type of motivation exhibited. Ridgeway (1982) found women to be almost as "influential" as men in mixed groups *if* they demonstrated motivation to assist the group in accomplishing its tasks. If women exhibited "self motivation" (i.e., unconcern for group goals and statement of individual concerns unrelated to group goals), they were likely to be both ignored and disliked (by males).

The fourth intervention strategy is manipulation of *numerical proportions.* Kanter (1977a, 1977b) reports that "balanced" groups are more positive for members of both sexes than "tilted" or "skewed" groups. Izraeli (1983, Note 1) found women's views of their influence on others to be greatly enhanced when a greater proportion of committee members was female.

*Women in All-Female Groups.* Little is said in the literature regarding interventions for overcoming unproductive interactional patterns in all-female groups. Carlock and Martin's (1977) finding that females in an all-female group experienced greater objective gains than those in a mixed group but subjectively enjoyed the group less suggests that group leaders may need to assist women in all-female groups to affirm the "legitimacy" and value of the group experience. Leader emphasis on humor, fun, positive affect, and the potential for objective benefits may counteract tendencies to view the group as unexciting or a waste of time.

In all-female task groups, leaders (experimenters) may wish to initiate discussions which differentiate leadership, influence, and power which are exploitative from those which instrumentally facilitate accomplishment of group goals. Rejection of such "male-identified" values as hierarchy, influence, and control has fused in some feminist groups with a rejection of a division of labor itself (cf. Baker, 1982). A consequence of this for all-female task groups may, as suggested by Eskilson and Wiley (1976), lead to objectively diminished success at task accomplishment. Explicit confrontation and resolution by women of their ambivalence towards females who "exercise influence" could possibly reduce the empirical occurrence of the "queen bee" syndrome, a topic frequently mentioned when "women vis-a-vis women" in work contexts are discussed (see Kanter, 1977a).

*Men in Mixed Groups.* Evidence on the effects of mixed groups for males is generally positive. Placing men with women in balanced groups influences men to become more personal (Aries, 1976) and less competitive and disagreeable (Piliavin & Martin, 1978). Encouragement by the experimenter of males to talk in mixed groups was found by Piliavin and Martin (1978) to produce fairly extreme stereotypical male behaviors (e.g., domination of interaction). Assuming a goal of down-playing gender roles and encouraging personal contributions unrelated to gender, this suggests that group leaders may wish to encourage males in mixed groups to listen rather than talk. Eskilson and Wiley (1976) found task groups with two males and one female to be unproductive because the males competed to gain the top leadership position and to impress the female. Overall, mixed groups, particularly balanced ones, are viewed as positive for males because they foster less stereotypical, more flexible, and more varied behaviors on their part (Yerby, 1975).

*Men in All-Male Groups.* Extant evidence on all-male task groups suggests they are both cooperative and effective. Leaders of all-male growth/discussion groups may, however, wish to affirm the appropriateness of intimacy, closeness, and self-relevatory norms in the group and to discourage excessive competition, disagreement, and conflict. The latter may also be useful in some all-male task groups.

## CONCLUSIONS

Present analyses reveal significant gaps in the recent literature on group sex composition. In particular, little research has been done on "non-task/work" groups, that is, discussion, growth, treatment, or therapy. The subtle yet powerful effects of sex composition may be mistakenly identified by participants as personal in origin, this omission is disturbing. The literature on task/work groups, although fairly extensive, suffers from numerous limitations. The majority of studies utilize university undergraduate students as subjects, raising question regarding the generalizability of observed effects. Similarly, studies of "real world work" groups are based primarily on survey data, raising internal validity questions regarding their results. With few exceptions, the effects of variables that may condition, or rival, those of sex composition have not been systematically examined (e.g., size of the group, see Patterson & Shaeffer, 1977; type of task assigned; whether group members are strangers or known to each other; and so forth). Finally, little attention has been paid to interventions in same sex groups which can mitigate effects which are viewed as undesirable. Status disadvantages suffered by females in task groups appear, from present literature, to surface not only in mixed groups but in all-female groups. Experimentation by both researchers and practitioners aimed at identifying interventions which can neutralize these effects would constitute a welcomed contribution to basic theoretical understanding of how status disadvantaged persons relate to each other in arenas from which they are normatively proscribed (e.g., women in task/work groups).

Considerable research confirms the conclusion that manipulation of "proportions" of men and women in mixed groups can improve the group experience for females. In particular, group leaders should avoid placement of a solo female in an otherwise male group. The addition of one more female significantly mitigates the negative effects which solos typically experience (see Frank & Katcher, 1977). On the other hand, a proportional "balance" of male and female members is not sufficient to erase *all* negative consequences for female participants in mixed groups. Additional interventions— such as legitimation, competency, motivational training, and so forth—are required for women to receive results and benefits equal to those of men in mixed groups.

## REFERENCE NOTES

1. Izraeli, D. N. Gender differences in self-reported influence among union officers. Paper presented at the American Psychological Association Symposium: Gender differences: the effects of status, power, and competence. Washington, D.C., August 24, 1982.
2. South, S. J., Bonjean, C. M., Markham, W. T., & Conder, J. Female labor participation and the organizational experiences of male workers. Unpublished manuscript, University of Houston, 1982.
3. Stacey, M. Women, power, and politics: Theoretical considerations. Paper presented at the Tenth World Congress of the International Sociological Association. Mexico City, D.F., Mexico, August 1982.
4. Szafran. R. F. Recruitment equity: accounting for organizational differences. Unpublished manuscript, University of Iowa, 1982.

## REFERENCES

Aries, E. Interaction patterns and themes of male, female and mixed groups. *Small Group Behavior,* 1976, *7,* 7-18.

Baker, A. J. The problems of authority in radical movement groups: A case study of lesbian-feminist organization. *The Journal of Applied Behavioral Science,* 1982, *18,* 323-341.

Bales, R. F., & Slater, P. Role differentiation in small decision making groups. In T. Parsons and R. F. Bales (eds.), *Family, socialization and interaction.* New York: Free Press, 1955.

Bartol, K. The effect of male versus female leaders on follower satisfaction and performance. *Journal of Business Research,* 1975, *3,* 33-42.

Berger, J., Cohen, B. P., & Zelditch, M. Status characteristics and social interaction. *American Sociological Review,* 1972, *37,* 241-255.

Berger, J., Fisek, H., Norman, R., & Zelditch, M. *Status characteristics, a social interaction: An expectation-states approach.* New York, N.Y.: Elsevier, 1977.

Berman, P. O'Nan, B., & Floyd, W. The double standard of aging and the social situation: Judgements of attractiveness of the middle-aged woman. *Sex Roles,* 1981, *7,* 87-95.

Bradley, P. Sex, competence and opinion deviation: An expectation states approach. *Communication Monographs,* 1980, *47,* 101-110.

Carlock, C. J., & Martin, P. Y. Sex composition and the intensive group experience. *Social Work,* 1977, *22,* 27-32.

Cohen, E. G., & Roper, S. S. Modification of interracial interaction disability: An application of status characteristics theory. *American Sociological Review,* 1972, *37,* 643-657.

Deaux, K. *The behavior of women and men.* Monterey, Calif.: Brooks Cole, 1976.

Eskilson, A., & Wiley, M. G. Sex composition and leadership in small groups. *Sociometry,* 1976, *39,* 183-194.

Fennell, M. L., Barchas, P., Cohen, E., McMahon, A., & Hildebrand, P. An alternative perspective on sex differences in organizational settings: The process of legitimation. *Sex Roles,* 1978, *4,* 589-604.

Frank, H. H., & Katcher, A. H. The qualities of leadership: How male medical students evaluate their female peers. *Human Relations,* 1977, *30,* 403-416.

Greene, L. R., Morrison, T. L., & Tischler, N. G. Aspects of identification in the large group. *The Journal of Social Psychology,* 1980, *111,* 91-97.

Izraeli, D. N. Sex effects or structural effects? an empirical test of Kanter's theory of proportions. *Social Forces,* 1983, *61.* Forthcoming.

Kanter, R. M. Some effects of proportions on group life: Skewed sex ratios and responses to token women. *American Journal of Sociology,* 1977a, *82,* 965-990.

Kanter, R. M. *Men and women of the corporation.* New York: Basic Books, 1977b.

Lockheed, M. E., & Hall, K. P. Conceptualizing sex as a status characteristic: Applications to leadership training strategies. *Journal of Social Issues,* 1976, *32,* 111-124.

Martin, P. Y., Harrison, D., & DiNitto, D. Advancement for women in hierarchical organizations: A multi-level analysis of problems and prospects. *Journal of Applied Behavioral Science,* 1983, *19.* Forthcoming.

Meeker, B. F., & Weitzel-O'Neill, P. A. Sex roles and interpersonal behavior in task-oriented groups. *American Sociological Review,* 1977, *42,* 91-105.

Patterson, M. L., & Schaffer, R. E. Effects of size and sex composition on interaction distance, participation and satisfaction in small groups. *Small Group Behavior,* 1977, *8,* 433-441.

Piliavin, J. A., & Martin, R. R. The effects of the sex composition of groups on style of social interaction. *Sex Roles,* 1978, *4,* 218-296.

Ridgeway, C. L. Status in groups: The importance of motivation. *American Sociological Review,* 1982, *47,* 76-88.

Ridgeway, C. L., & Jacobson, C. K. Sources of status and influence in all-female and mixed-sex groups. *The Sociological Quarterly,* 1977, Summer, 413-425.

Ruble, D., & Higgins, E. T. Effects of group sex composition on self-presentation and sex-typing. *Journal of Social Issues,* 1976, *32,* 125-132.

Shomer, R. W., & Centers, R. Differences in attitudinal responses under conditions of implicitly manipulated group salience. *Journal of Personality and Social Psychology,* 1970, *15,* 125-132.

South, S. J., Bonjean, C. M., Markham, W. T., & Conder, J. Social structure and intergroup interaction. *American Sociological Review,* 1982, *47,* 587-599.

Spangler, E., Gordon, M. A., & Pipkin, R. M. Token women: An empirical test of Kanter's hypothesis. *American Journal of Sociology,* 1978, *84,* 160-170.

Thune, E. S., Manderscheid, R. W., & Silbergeld, S. Status or sex roles as determinants of interaction patterns in small mixed-groups. *The Journal of Social Psychology,* 1980, *112,* 51-65.

Webster, M., & Driskell, J. E. Status generalization: A review and some new data. *American Sociological Review,* 1978, *43,* 220-236.

Wiley, M., & Eskilson, A. Coping in the corporation: Sex role constraints. *Journal of Applied Social Psychology,* 1982, *12,* 1-11.

Wolman, C., & Frank, H. The solo woman in a professional peer group. *American Journal of Orthopsychiatry,* 1975, *41,* 164-170.

Yerby, J. Attitude, task, and sex composition as variables affecting female leadership in small problem solving groups. *Speech Monographs,* 1975, *42,* 160-168.

# WOMEN LEADERS IN SMALL GROUPS: SOCIAL-PSYCHOLOGICAL, PSYCHODYNAMIC, AND INTERACTIONAL PERSPECTIVES

These two papers present different, but complementary perspectives for understanding the existing evidence about the impact of women group leaders. In the first, Beth Glover Reed posits that women leaders are perceived to be both role and status incongruent. Group members are often confused and upset by these inconsistencies which disrupt their expectations, the usual ways that groups form and operate, and even the balance of power and related role expectations between women and men in the group.

Teresa Bernardez then reviews psychodynamic and interactional perspectives on the origins and functions of both men's and women's unconscious fears of female power and dominance. She describes the repressed stereotype of the vengeful or totally selfless mother and how a woman leader's behavior can either arouse irrational reactions or contain them. Gender socialization for both genders further influences how women and men react to women leaders and to each other in groups with women leaders.

## CALL FOR PAPERS

Special Edition of *Social Work with Groups:* "Time-Limited Groups."

Under the Dual Guest Editorship of A.S. Alissi and Max Casper.

You are invited to submit manuscripts dealing with different aspects of social group work practice, theory and research on time-limited group experiences:

* The use of short-term frames in practice
* The single session group experience
* On-going group structures with changing memberships
* Differential use of skills, techniques and methods in long-term, short-term and single session groups

Manuscript is due by December 1, 1983.

Manuscripts may be submitted to the Guest Editors or to the Editors of *Social Work with Groups.* Please refer to Instructions for Authors.

Albert S. Alissi, University of Connecticut, School of Social Work, Greater Hartford Campus, West Hartford, Conn. 06117.

Max Casper, Syracuse University, School of Social Work, Brockway Hall, Syracuse, New York 13210.

# Women Leaders in Small Groups: Social-Psychological Perspectives and Strategies

Beth Glover Reed

Most small group research and theory have been derived from leaderless groups or groups with men leaders. Relatively recently, researchers and practitioners have begun to examine the leadership behaviors of men compared to women; group member reactions to, and perceptions of, women leaders; and the ways that relationships among members, group development, norms and structure may be influenced by a group leader's gender.

In this paper and the one that follows, we will briefly review some of the research results and theories that have been posited to account for the findings. We will also identify some ways that women leaders can minimize some of the negative reactions to their leadership and take advantage of the opportunities to promote growth, learning and new knowledge.

The research results are complex and sometimes contradictory. As yet, there has been no program of research that has systematically varied leader gender in different types of groups and situations. Size, composition, and task have varied widely in studies to date. As a result, we do not yet know how regularly and under what circumstances the effects I will describe occur. Some of them may also be modified as societal conceptions of gender change and as women leaders become more common.

Despite this uncertainty, the gender of its leader clearly affects a group, and group workers need to consider the implications of our knowledge thus far in composing, planning, implementing, and

Beth Glover Reed is Associate Professor, School of Social Work, University of Michigan, 1065 Frieze Building, Ann Arbor, MI 48109.

evaluating groups. This knowledge also should be incorporated into group work education programs, in-service training, and supervision, or women group workers will be only partially prepared for what they will encounter as group leaders (Reed, 1981).

The majority of studies find that men and women leaders usually behave in similar ways, but that women are often perceived and reacted to differently from men, usually more negatively. Women-led groups are often reported to be more stressful and confusing for both members and leader (although the gender of member, the gender composition of the group, its size and task interact with these perceptions and reactions). There is also some evidence that relationships among members, group development, and even its structural characteristics are affected by the gender of its leader.

## THEORETICAL PERSPECTIVES

### Actuarial Prejudice and Role Incongruence

Kiesler (1975) discusses actuarial prejudice in her review of some of the evidence about society's generally negative biases about women's abilities and their "proper" place in life. Although the widespread conceptions about masculine and feminine behaviors and roles are not all negative (cf., Broverman, Vogel, Broverman, Clarkson, & Rosenkrantz, 1972; Bem, 1974), many views of women are incompatible with conceptions of competent leadership. Thus, behaviors expected of leaders would be viewed as role discrepant when exhibited by women and are evaluated differently, often more negatively, than the same behaviors exhibited by men. A woman leader is also likely to be sent conflicting messages about how members expect her to behave (leaderlike, but feminine) and, since many of these are incompatible, her inability to meet all of these expectations can lead to dissatisfaction with her performance.

Laws (1975) proposes that a woman who occupies a role that is not consistent with women's socially defined roles and status is doubly deviant. She deviates as do all women from the dominant culture of the society because she is not male, and deviates from female culture by not being appropriately female. Thus, a woman leader is likely to face the dilemmas of the token described by Kanter (1977a, 1977b, 1977c), Kanter and Stein (1980). A person is usually described as a token when members of a social category she represents (in this case, female) are greatly outnumbered in a group or organization. Even when she is not the only woman in a group, as leader, a woman occupies a role more commonly occupied by men, and is thus different from the other women.

In a token situation, the behavior of the token is usually scrutinized carefully, differences between that person and other members are exaggerated, and the person may be isolated from other members. Kanter has identified some of the stereotypes commonly assigned to token women (earth mother, sex object, mascot, and iron maiden), all of which are limiting.

Even if token dynamics do not contribute to group members' reactions to women leaders, such stereotyping is likely, especially if group members have had little experience with women in leadership roles. Especially when a situation is new, ambiguous or stressful, people tend to rely on past experience and stereotypes to guide their behavior; they may well behave as if the woman leader is occupying some other female role with which they have more experience (wife, daughter, sister, sexual partner, or friend).

## Status Incongruence

Another interpretation arises from the concepts of diffuse status characteristics and associated role expectations (Berger, Cohen, & Fisek, 1974; Berger, Cohen, & Zelditch, 1972; Berger, Fisek, Norman, & Zelditch, 1977). The different role expectations associated with *masculine* and *feminine* are also associated with different status rankings within the larger culture; male is the more valued state. Thus, a woman occupying a leadership role is not only role-incongruent; she is also status-incongruent. She simultaneously occupies (at least) two roles: female, which is the lower status of gender, and leader, which is a higher status position than member. Gender is a basic organizing concept within the culture so expectations related to it are pervasive and affect our assumptions and perceptions across a wide range of situations. *Leader* is more likely to be an earned or achieved status with expectations limited primarily to the situation in which one is to lead.

Similar to role incongruence, status incongruence leads to conflicting expectations and confusion about how to interact with the person whose status characteristics are inconsistent. It is often stressful both for the woman in the position and for those who must interact with her. Group members may try to find ways to avoid the situation or the person, and are likely to maintain consistency among the different levels of status by averaging them or distorting information about one or the other position. Since gender is the more diffuse characteristic, they are likely to discount a woman's leadership abilities and credentials first in order to maintain their assumptions about women having lower status. They may also act as if someone else is the leader, try to take over the leadership themselves, or behave as if the group has no leader. If these strategies are unsuccessful because her leadership is inescapable or because she is clearly a competent leader, they may then try to ignore her gender. If that too fails, then members have to adjust their perceptions that women have less value than men, which is likely to lead to a re-evaluation of many gender-related assumptions and behaviors.

## IMPLICATIONS FOR WOMEN GROUP LEADERS

All of the theories and much of the available data suggest that groups with women leaders are likely to be, at minimum, more confusing for both members and leader. Women leaders are less familiar to the leader, to members, and in the literature. Developing a cohesive, productive group is less likely if members try to avoid a woman leader or the group situation. Devaluing her leadership abilities or acting as if she is occupying other female roles in relation to them will make it difficult for her to use her skills optimally. In some groups, this can lead to excessive anxiety that potentially threatening dynamics cannot be controlled; in others it may lead to dependency behaviors and ambivalent reliance on the leader for structure and direction; in still others, it can lead to rebellion and an inability to work together. The often uncomfortable and frustrating early stages of group formation and developing norms and procedures may be greatly prolonged since these reactions to the woman leader can interfere with clarifying leadership and power issues and make norm development more complex.

The re-evaluation of gender as a status characteristic would also disrupt the role expectations associated with each gender and shift the usual power balance between men and women. While these shifts can be confusing and even threatening for members, especially if they do not understand what is happening, they also provide enormous opportunities for growth and learning among members. While groups with men leaders largely reinforce stereotypic gender behaviors and perceptions, those with women leaders can open up alternative options for both genders (Mayes, 1979; Reed, 1979).

These dynamics can be controlled and may not be noticed in groups with concrete tasks or a lot of structure, but they may emerge at times of stress or change. Women group workers and those who supervise them must be aware of the ways in which women-led groups can be different from those led by men. They must also consider some of the ways that potential problems can be contained and possible benefits optimized. In the next section, I will discuss some of these ways.

## SPECIFIC SUGGESTIONS

Many of the dynamics described here are not simply problems that can be solved if a leader has enough knowledge and skills. Because of the lack of attention to gender in group leadership training programs, many women assume that they somehow "aren't doing it right" when groups they lead are different from those described in the literature. The effects of gender are very powerful, influencing groups even in the absence of interaction (Ruble & Higgens, 1976) and affecting many aspects, including even the amount of space allocated to each member (Biesen & McClaren, 1976). Traditional group knowledge and group skills are certainly necessary, but will not remove the influence of leader gender on the group. Simply understanding this will free many women to explore alternative explanations and strategies for the situations they encounter in groups they lead.

Leader style and behaviors are fraught with dilemmas for the woman wishing to work with groups. If she behaves in ways that reduce role incongruence (i.e., develop a more "feminine" leadership style), her behavior is likely to remind members of her lower gender status and perpetuate status incongruence. On the other hand, a more reciprocating leadership style seems to decrease discomfort in groups with women leaders but doesn't seem to decrease discomfort in groups with women leaders but doesn't seem to make much difference in groups with men leaders (Wright, 1976). Particular styles and characteristics may be more likely to elicit some female stereotypes (e.g., mother or sex object). A woman leader may be tempted to behave inconsistently trying to respond to different expectations and needs within the group. Because of the increased ambivalence and confusion in her groups, she is likely to get more distorted feedback than a man leader would about how she is perceived and what members think and feel about the group and its accomplishments.

For all these reasons, it is especially important that women group workers understand how others react to them in interpersonal situations, and that they have clear well-developed communication skills, so that they can begin to sort out real feedback about behaviors they should modify, from stereotypes and distortions related to their gender. The complexity of women-led groups is confusing for their leaders too, and getting regular, well-informed supervision or consultation can be crucial if a leader is to think clearly about the group. Support and assistance in analyzing group sessions will be very important if gender-related dynamics become strong.

Whenever possible, a woman leader should be clear and explicit abut her expectations and why she is behaving as she is. Such clarity minimizes the risk of unhelpful stereotyping and can help contain anxiety and confusion.

In some cases, it may be important to make sure a leader's authority is clear and legitimate. This will increase the leader's status, but can also lead to further unrealistic expectations. Because of the different behavioral standards that we use to evaluate men and women, a highly credentialed woman is often rated as *more* competent than a man with similar credentials and performance (e.g., Taynor & Deaux, 1973), and members may then continue to expect more of her.

One of the most useful things that leaders of either gender can do is to include education about gender and its effects in their work with groups. In some task groups, this may not be appropriate, but may be necessary even in work groups if reactions to the leader's gender interfere with the group's effectiveness. The knowledge presented in many of the papers in this collection can help members understand how they are feeling and reacting and will give them the cognitive tools they will need to learn from, or cope with, the situation. Education about the possible effects of leader gender at the time a woman assumes a leadership role can help prevent problematic gender-related dynamics from developing, and will make them easier to discuss if they occur. In groups with therapeutic or learning goals, having a woman leader can open up whole new areas of learning and growth for members with the inclusion of some of this educational content.

Finally, the use of co-leadership models in different kinds of groups must be examined. Many group training programs rely heavily on co-leadership experiences, with neophyte group workers paired with more experienced workers and then with peers, for supervision and support. In my case, I had been doing group work extensively for three years, and had trained a number of junior people before I ever had occasion to run a group by myself. In some ways this was fortunate since by that time in my training I knew there was something different about the group and not with me. On the other hand, all of the co-leadership experience had only partially prepared me for what I experience leading a group alone. There is some evidence, in fact, that male-female co-leadership situations may perpetuate gender-stereotypic behaviors in groups, even when both leaders are behaving in nonstereotypic ways for their gender. Members commonly misattribute particular behaviors to the leader of the gender associated with that behavior. Even female-female pairing may elicit stereotyping, with one perceived as more "masculine" and one, more "feminine."

This evidence suggests that groups with women leaders, although not always pleasant, may be among the best ways to facilitate learning about gender and its effects—in individuals and in social situations. There are also great opportunities to add to the literature.

## REFERENCES

Bem, S. L. The measurement of psychological androgeny. *Journal of Consulting and Clinical Psychology*, 1974, *42*, 155-162.

Berger, J., Cohen, B. P. & Zelditch, M., Jr. Status characteristics and social interaction. *American Sociological Review*, 1972, *37*, 241-255.

Berger, J., Cohen, T. L., & Fisek, M. H. (Eds.) *Expectation stages theory: A theoretical research program.* Cambridge, MA: Winthrop, 1974.

Berger, J., Fisek, M. H., Norman, R. Z. & Zelditch, M., Jr. *Status characteristics and social interaction: An expectation-states approach.* New York: Elsevier, 1977.

Broverman, I. K., Vogel, S. R., Broverman, D. M., Clarkson, R. E., & Rosenkrantz, P. S. Sex role stereotypes: A current appraisal. *Journal of Social Issues*, 1972, *28*(2), 59-78.

Giesen, M. & McClaren, H. A. Discussion, distance and sex: Changes in impressions and attraction during small group interactions. *Sociometry*, 1976, *39*(1), 60-70.

Kanter, R. M. *Men and women of the corporation.* New York: Basic Books, 1977(a).

Kanter, R. M. Some effects of proportions in group life: Skewed sex ratios and responses to token women. *American Journal of Sociology*, 1977(b), *82*, 965-990.

Kanter, R. M. Women in organizations: Sex roles, group dynamics, and change strategies. In A. Sargent (Ed.), *Beyond Sex Roles.* St. Paul, Minn.: West Publishing Co., 1977(c), 371-386.

Kanter, R. M. & Stein, B. A. *The tale of "O": On being different in an organization.* New York: Harper & Row, 1980.

Laws, J. L. The psychology of tokenism: An analysis. *Sex Roles*, 1975, *1*, 51-67.

Kiesler, S. B. Actuarial prejudice towards women and its implications. *Journal of Applied Social Psychology,* 1975, *5,* 201-216.

Mayes, S. S. Women in positions of authority: A case study of changing sex roles. *Signs: Journal of Women in Culture and Society,* 1979, *4,* 556-568.

Reed, B. G. Differential reactions by male and female group members in the presence of male or female authority figures (Doctoral Dissertation, University of Cincinnati, 1979). *Dissertation Abstracts International,* 1980 (University Microfilms No. 8002133).

Reed, B. G. Gender issues in training group leaders. *Journal for Specialists in Group Work,* *6*(3), 1981, 161-171.

Ruble, D. N. & Higgins, E. T. Effects of group sex composition on self-presentation and sex-typing. *Journal of Social Issues,* 1976, *32*(3), 125-132.

Taynor, J., & Deaux, K. When women are more deserving than men: Equity, attribution, and perceived sex differences. *Journal of Personality and Social Psychology,* 1973, *20,* 360-367.

Wright, F. The effects of style and sex of consultants in self-study groups. *Small Group Behavior,* 1976, *7,* 443-456.

# Women in Authority: Psychodynamic and Interactional Aspects

Teresa Bernardez

Femininity and power are attributes that have been seen as incompatible with one another in this culture. To understand the pervasiveness of the fear of female power and the attendant attitudes towards women in authority, the social context and the intrapsychic and interactional forces at work in men and women have to be examined in their interrelations.

The prevalent view of the culture has been that the female sex is inferior to the male and less competent to exercise functions socially assigned to males. The ubiquitousness of these views and the way they are structured in the social world have been amply documented (Carmen, Russo, & Miller, 1981). It stands to reason then, that when a female assumes a position of power and is hierarchically superior to the male, she is bound to evoke responses that denote the incongruity between the actual situation and the beliefs of the subordinate. But the irrationality of the responses, the intense affective charge with which they are colored and the character of the criticism that females in leadership frequently evoke, need greater analysis to make them intelligible. I will propose a set of hypothesis using observations of the behavior of men and women in groups and organizations, clarifying the role of male and female socialization in the complex interactions of both sexes with women in leadership

Teresa Bernardez is Professor in Psychiatry, Department of Psychiatry, College of Osteopathic Medicine and College of Human Medicine, Michigan State University, A 236 E. Fee, Lansing, MI 48824.

positions and the effect on women given their deviant status as authorities.


## UNCONSCIOUS FEAR OF FEMALE POWER AND DOMINANCE

The phenomenon of "status incongruence" (Reed, this volume) is further fueled in the case of women in power by the males' unconscious fear of female power and dominance and by the cultural prohibitions on males of experiences that denote submission, passivity, and dependence. Dinnerstein (1977) has paid attention to the fear of female power in the way heterosexual relations are structured. Bernardez (1978) has commented on the influence that the repressed stereotype of the vengeful mother exercises in inhibiting aggressive behavior in the female and in sensitizing males to female anger and criticism. Lerner (1974) describes a similar origin of the envy of the male and his consequent devaluation of the female.

The tendency to devalue women and to deny or ignore their competence has, therefore, a number of determinants in men: the superiority of the dominant class and/or of any member of that class is put into question if the ability and competence of the woman is obvious and leads her to positions of power. Some men react as if they had been humiliated when a woman demonstrates her excellence over them. That is why it is frequent to find among women, the tendency to minimize their abilities and to diminish their visibility. Kanter (1977) comments on the fear of retaliation in women whose excellence may make "the dominants look bad." This adaptive response in women has been reinforced in their socialization: women are permitted to exhibit only their physical attributes but there are strong prohibitions about "showing off" in areas where they may compete with men. Thus, we have often an interactional pattern that maintains in abeyance the dread of female power—men needing to devalue women and ignore their abilities, and women making themselves invisible in obedience with the injunctions of their socialization and to avoid retaliation from men.

The model of female authority is a primitive and irrational one, since it is not just the mother of childhood (and in subsequent years the female teacher) but the idealized and feared image of her, that is maintained out of awareness. The scarcity of women leaders in public life and the lack of models of feminine authority in the adult lives of individuals does not permit us to edit and review these early versions of interactions with females in power.

Chodorow (1982) has focused attention on the idealized mother in the fantasy of the perfect mother, present potentially in each woman. The aspects of this fantasy that have relevance for the study of interactions of men and women with female authorities are (1) her selflessness: she has no needs of her own, she exists for others; (2) her total acceptance: she loves and accepts under all circumstances; (3) her abnegation; (4) her lack of aggression and criticism; and (5) her nurturance.

Female leaders unwittingly arouse these expectations in members of their groups and organizations. When their behavior runs counter to this ideal version (i.e., when dissatisfied, critical, or rejecting) and/or when the group/institution has characteristics that encourage regression (i.e., unclear role definition, unclear delineation of tasks, structureless groups, contradictory expectations) irrational and intense anger and criticism can befall her. The personal characteristics of the woman leader can either minimize or exaggerate the response but do not totally prevent it.

Mayes (1979) describes these reactions in males and subsequent female reactions caused in part by their fear of loss of the males' love. But females too, tend to reveal the presence of potent feelings and irrational expectations when the group structure and the leader's behavior permits its open exposure. In all female groups (Bernardez, 1978) this phenomenon has been explored for therapeutic purposes. The female members move back and forth from idealization of the leader with expectations for nurturance, acceptance and empowerment to rejection and anger because the leader does not provide for them. The competition with the powerful female, the wish to separate and differentiate from her and the desire to fuse with her and regain a presumed state of power and bliss are powerful forces in the female-female dyad. Unlike men, women have had to contend with their second-class status. They usually blame mother for it and unless they have had the opportunity to work through experiences of disappointment and loss with their mothers or later substitutes, feelings of anger at the injustice and betrayal they have experienced are expressed in situations that evoke the original one.

In mixed groups—as Mayes and Kanter comment on—women react to the female leader *in context with the males' response* and their own expectations and fears of their relations with males. It is precisely in mixed groups where women may need to demonstrate that they are not like the leader by rejecting her and criticizing her in excess.

## THE INFLUENCE OF GENDER SOCIALIZATION

These situations that reveal the need of the members to diminish the presumed power of the female leader, to dissuade her from continuing to exercise authority and to deter her from assuming control of the group can be understood further by looking at the socialization of the male and at the cultural prohibition to identify with females. In a previous work (Bernardez, 1983) I have contended that many males in this culture are divorced from aspects of themselves, particularly those that are early identifications with the maternal object, by a complex process of counter-identification in response to the culture's injunction against being female-like.

This negative identification with women places men in a continuous struggle with aspects of themselves that need to be warded off, and in many cases, the splitting of those aspects and their projection onto women permit a temporary equilibrium. The male thus controls in the female aspects of himself that he fears and devalues. The domination of women is encouraged by the culture, but its strength comes from the need of males to control and dominate the female-self in themselves. This defense is threatened when a woman in power appears to have control. Not only is the male not in control of the satisfaction of his dependency needs but he may fear the loss of control of aspects of himself that are frequently projected onto women. A woman in control is thus experienced by males in this situation as controlling them, dominating them, and forcing upon them behaviors that have highly negative value for them: passivity, submissiveness, compliance, dependency.

In turn, the female is reared with a counter-fear: that of dominance and control of the male. As long as the sexes operate within the limits of these unconscious injunctions they can maintain a fairly harmonious and complementary relationship but when the female deviates from the norm and furthermore, places herself in precisely the most threatening position, she is seen as disrupting the protection erected against a number of disturbing feelings and unresolved conflicts.

If in addition, we posit that the socialization of women also tends to instruct them carefully against disrupting this order and against expressing aggressiveness, particularly toward males, we can understand the paralyzing and distressing effects that the intense and bitter criticism of male subordinates have on women. Leaders who are vulnerable to this aggression (i.e., showing self-injury or withdrawal) appear to generate more of it. The female authority models who appear to meet the test with more success are those who are capable of firm benevolence: not bothered by the aggression and who can protect themselves from it and are capable of greater detachment, neutrality and objectivity. The female leader's ability to *contain the aggression* without retaliation, helplessness or expression of intense affect in return, seems to be able to permit the group eventual recognition of more reality oriented perceptions of her power and more accurate readings of her capacities and goals.

If we use Bion's (1960) theories about the underlying expectations in his "basic assumption groups" we could say that dependency and fight-flight groups are readily recognized in the irrational eruption of affect in the female-led groups. Often enough, nurturing and supportive, self-effacing female authorities are given a good chance to lead harmonious groups. In this case, although the female is in power, she appears to use it totally for the benefit of the members and she portrays reassuringly the characteristics of the idealized mother image. Keeping within these limits, lack of sexual attractiveness is seen as an asset: sexual attraction in association with power in females carries a potential threat.

This does not mean that women who are perceived as the maternal stereotypes are the ones who can hope to elicit cooperation and creativity. Many women in authority with differing characteristics have been able to introduce change and to alter power-related interactions in their own systems with great success. The more reality-centered the group and the more able the leader to contain the aggression of the group and deal with the irrationality, firmly but neutrally, the less likely that the groups effectiveness will be impaired. In some instances, it is precisely a female leader who can produce the desired change. Much of the socialization of women tends to be helpful when they are in leadership roles since women have greater interpersonal skills, they tend to delegate and run more open and democratic systems and are more likely to share power (Neuse, 1978).

## WOMEN AS SOURCES OF MORAL POWER

Among the archetypal characteristics of the idealized mother image is the capacity to make moral judgements, to be beyond good and evil, to be the omniscient judge. Mothers are the first superegos and ego-ideals against whom we struggle for the satisfaction of our needs and impulses. They are the antecedents of our consciences.

Perhaps because of their absence in public life, women tend to be viewed as less apt to be corrupted by power and more inclined to be ethical than men. When a woman in authority disagrees with the norms established by the dominants, her disagreement is often perceived as an indictment. In male dominated environments, it is not infrequent that the group accepts norms that are convenient but not always ethical. The members avoid responsibility to relying on group consensus but if the woman (the deviant member) disagrees with the state of affairs, her attitude is perceived as one of moral criticism. In addition to the phenomenon of group solidarity (Kanter, 1977) what is aroused here is the expectation of the moral judgement of the female particularly because the guilt felt by the members about their own behavior—assuaged until then by the validation of the group—and the self-reproach that generates it is projected onto the woman and defended against by righteous indignation. Since males tend to be socialized to ward off affects that induce passivity, helplessness and dependence, they are prone to react with defensive anger in situations which arouse such emotions. The anger can be very intense and may be unconsciously used to silence the expected negative judgement from the female.

Although women in leadership roles may be castigated for their perceived disapproval, they may also serve to enhance the group's desire to transform itself and achieve a higher integration. The specific ingredients that women and other minorities have to offer are linked with aspects that are devalued by the dominant culture but that paradoxically must be integrated to achieve increasing harmony and creativity. An instance of this is the humanization of technocratic institutions and the democratization of hierarchical organizations when women enter them in greater numbers.

## REFERENCES

Bernardez, T. Women and anger: Conflicts with aggression in contemporary women. *J. of the AMWA*, Vol. 33:5:215-219, 1978.

Bernardez, T. Women's groups: A feminist perspective on the treatment of women. Chapter in *Changing Approaches to the Psychotherapies,* Grayson and Lowe, Spectrum Pub. Inc., pp: 55-67, 1978.

Bernardez, T. The female therapist in relation to male roles. In *Men in Transition: Theory and Therapy,* Solomon and Levy (eds.), Plenum Pub., 1982.

Carmen, E., Russo, N. and Miller J. Inequality and women's mental health: An overview. *Am. J. Psychiatry, 138*(10), 1981.

Chodorow, N. and Contratto, S. The fantasy of the perfect mother. In *Rethinking the Family.* B. Thorne (ed.), Longman, NY, pp: 54-75, 1982.

Dinnerstein, D. *The Mermaid and the Minotaur.* Harper and Row, NY, 1977.

Kanter, R. M. Some effects of proportions on group life: Skewed sex ratios and responses to token women. *Am. J. Sociology, 85*(5), 965-990, 1977.

Lerner, H. Early origins of envy and the devaluation of women: Implications for sex role stereotypes. *Bulletin of the Menninger Clinic, 38*(6), 1974.

Mayes, S. Women in positions of authority: A case study of changing sex roles. *Signs, 4*(3), 556-568, 1979.

Neuse, S. M. Professionalism and authority: Women in public service. *Public Administration Review, 38,* 436-441, 1978.

# Gender Issues Related
# to Group Social Skills Training

Eileen Gambrill
Cheryl A. Richey

**ABSTRACT.** Social skills training helps group members to develop ways to behave competently in specific interpersonal situations. This paper identifies gender related issues in such training and describes a non-sexist response to them. Some of the issues dealt with are the status considerations women face in assuming many roles, the gender biases in tools used to assess social skills, and the way gender affects cognitive and emotional variables related to such skills. Another issue discussed is that in discriminatory situations women, in particular, should be helped to change such situations or to resist their detrimental effects. Workers must be helped to recognize and change their own biases in these respects.

The aim of social skills training is to offer people more effective ways of behaving in specific interpersonal situations. Social skills training is a competency based approach to social interaction in contrast to a deficiency based approach. Emphasis is placed upon increasing people's ability to *construct competencies* (Mischel, 1981) and in offering them additional skills. Ineffective social skills have been implicated in a wide range of presenting concerns including relationship discord, sexual dysfunctions, depression, aggressive reactions, substance abuse, speech anxiety, shyness, and unemployment (Gambrill, 1977; McFall, 1982). This article discusses gender issues as they relate to group social skills training.

The term social skills training is gradually supplanting the term assertion training. The aim of assertion training, which has been especially popular with women, is to increase effective interper-

Eileen Gambrill is a professor at the School of Social Welfare at the University of California, Berkeley, California and Cheryl A. Richey is an Associate Professor at the School of Social Work at the University of Washington, Seattle, Washington. Professor Gambrill's mailing address for reprint requests is 120 Haveland Hall, Berkeley, CA 94720.

sonal skills, especially those which encourage participants to express their preferences so that others take these into account (see for example Alberti & Emmons, 1982; Jakubowski & Lange, 1978). Assertive behavior, by definition, refers to socially effective behavior. Passive and aggressive behavior refer to two ways in which social behavior may be ineffective (allowing rights to be ignored, or, the hostile expression of preference in a way that ignores the rights of others).

Gender biases may intrude at all stages of social skills or assertion training including planning group composition, deciding upon the purposes of the group, gathering assessment information, selecting intervention plans, and deciding how to maintain gains. Even people who work hard to avoid gender biases can easily slip into them. Examples are offered in the following sections together with suggestions for avoiding these.

## DEFINITIONAL, THEORETICAL, AND EMPIRICAL CONSIDERATIONS

A discussion of gender and social skills is complex since social skills encompass the broad general area of interpersonal behavior, and because the concept of gender cannot be discussed intelligently without considering related concepts of gender identity, sexual orientation, sex roles, and gender differences. The most satisfying empirical and theoretical view of social behavior attends to cognitions and emotions as well as to overt behavior (e.g., Argyle, Furnham, & Graham, 1981; Trower, 1982). Within this view, the person is not only an agent of action but a "watcher, commentator, and critic as well" (Trower, 1982, p. 412). There is, for example, increasing evidence that thoughts influence the quality of social behavior (Alden & Cappe, 1981; Eisler, Frederiksen, & Peterson, 1978; Glass & Merluzzi, 1981).

This process model of social skills includes attention to cognitive, physiological and overt behaviors. These components, including appropriate goals and plans, and attention to feedback from others, correspond to ways in which social behavior can be deficient (Furnham & Argyle, 1981). Accurate perception and translation of social cues is required. Competent social behavior also requires knowledge of the rules about what may and may not be done in specific situations in relation to the pursuit of goals; what may be effective in one situation may not be in another. Other components of competent social behavior include skill in taking the role of the other, effective verbal and non-verbal behaviors, appropriate self-presentation, and emotion management skills.

Important distinctions can be made among social skills, social skill, social competence, and social performance (Trower, 1982). *Social skills* refer to the components that people use in social interaction such as duration of eye contact, posture, and verbal statements. Trower defines *social skill* as "the process of generating skilled behavior directed toward a goal" (p. 418), *social competence* as the possession of the capability to generate skilled behavior," and *social performance* as the "actual production of skilled behavior in specific situations" (p. 419). The distinction between "social skills" and "social skill" is important since a man or woman may have effective social skills but these may be spoiled by inappropriate goals, incomplete plans, faulty processing of feedback from others, or inaccurate timing of response.

Distinctions must be made among the terms gender, gender identity, sex roles, and sexual orientation (see Garvin & Reed, this volume).

Another important concept related to but not synonymous with gender is status or power. Differences in social status or social power cut across gender, but in our society, characteristics of lower status individuals are more likely to be associated with *feminine* characteristics, since women as a group are afforded less status than men as a group. Thus, differences between men and women may be attributed erroneously to gender differences when actually the difference is a reflection of status inequities (lower status males behave with higher status males as women behave with men). As Crosby and others (1981) point out, "most of the asymmetries between women's and men's speech mirror asymmetries between the speech of low status individuals and high status individuals (p. 154).

## OFFERING A NON-SEXIST GROUP ENVIRONMENT

Social skills training is often conducted in a group setting. Trainers must be aware of stereotypes they hold and how these may influence their effectiveness as well as the accuracy of information they possess about gender differences. Since women comprise the majority of consumers of social services, it is especially important that trainers be aware of stereotypes they hold about women. The literature indicates that male workers must be especially careful about their gender biases since they are more likely to have them compared to women and they are less likely to be informed about women (Sherman, Koufacos, & Kenworthy, 1978). Liberalness of attitude is not necessarily matched by accurate information about women (Sherman, Koufacos, & Kenworthy, 1978). The influence of stereotypes on perception at an unconscious level is supported by the finding that "a woman at the head of a mixed-sex group was not viewed as more leaderlike by feminists, females, or those who were androgenous than by nonfeminists, males, or the sex typed" (Porter & Geis, 1981, p. 53).

Stereotypes are maintained in part by our language habits. Women tend to be defined in relational terms (for example, in relation to their husbands), whereas men are often referred to in occupational terms (Thorne & Henley, 1975). The prevalence of "he" rather than "she" in use of pronouns is ubiquitous. It is important that social skills trainers offer clients a non-sexist environment, one characteristic of which is use of non-sexist language. Trainers should be sure to balance examples used between men and women, to attend to women as often as men in mixed gender groups, to support deviations from dysfunctional sex role behavior such as elaborated opinion statements by women and the expression of feelings by men. Co-leading a group with a trainer of another gender may be helpful in catching and examining stereotypes. Information concerning sex bias in research will help trainers to be cautious in accepting conclusions drawn (Grady, 1981). Acquiring knowledge about gender differences is easier than examining stereotypes. Appropriate journal articles or books can be consulted and information noted that is especially germane to particular kinds of social skill training groups (e.g., Mayo & Henley, 1981).

Process variables should be an important consideration in deciding upon group composition (see Martin & Shanahan, this volume). Participation of people who do not conform to stereotypes held as well as people who can describe the unpleasant effects of being stereotyped may facilitate a shift away from stereotypes.

## ASSESSMENT CONSIDERATIONS

Careful assessment is necessary to identify relevant situations, to determine whether required skills are available, to find out whether there are discrimination problems in relation to when behaviors can most profitably be displayed, and to determine whether negative thoughts or emotions such as anxiety or anger interfere with effective behavior (Gambrill, 1977). It is thus important not only to identify the person's ability to construct effective behavior but also to identify factors that may interfere with their expression, such as negative expectations. Assessment tasks that are related to gender considerations include selection of sources of assessment information, selection of goals, selection of progress indicators, and selection of intervention focus. Ignorance of gender and status differences, and confusions among gender, gender identity, sexual orientation, and sex-role stereotypes, may result in serious decision errors by social workers who conduct social skill or assertion training groups. For example, trainers may use inappropriate standards to judge the effectiveness of different behaviors. Decision errors will result in lost opportunities to help clients achieve valued goals. Decision errors can also result in the faulty imposition of labels, including *false positives* (labeling a person as having a problem when she does not) as well as *false negatives* (assuming a person does not have a concern when she does). The former may unnecessarily stigmatize the individual and the latter may interfere with effective pursuit of goals.

## Selecting Sources of Assessment Information

A variety of sources of assessment information are available including self-report in the interview, observation in analogue, interview, or real-life situations, self-monitoring, and self-reported responses on standardized paper and pencil measures. Gathering assessment information from several sources is important because social skill difficulties may involve affective and cognitive, as well as behavioral response systems. Questionnaires have several disadvantages which require attention from the trainer concerned about gender issues in assessment. People may respond to questions in ways they believe are socially desirable. For example, women who scored high on social desirability also tended to describe themselves as more assertive and less anxious on the Assertion Inventory (Gambrill & Richey, 1975) than they actually appeared in analogue role-play situations (Kiecolt & McGrath, 1979). Another disadvantage of self-report questionnaires concerning social behavior is that general rather than specific information about social behavior is usually collected. This may account for the lack of consistency with which gender differences are found on such measures.

*Self-monitoring* is frequently used in social skills training programs to gather assessment information and to monitor progress.
For example, group members interested in increasing their social
contacts may keep track of how many conversations they initiate
each week (a conversation being defined as an interchange lasting
three minutes or more), their enjoyment and discomfort levels in
each interaction, and their degree of satisfaction with goal attainment (Gambrill & Richey, in press). The use of self-monitoring to
gather information places more control over the counseling process
in the hands of consumers, whether men or women. Thus, the
potential for gender biases imposed by trainers who rely solely on
standardized measures, their own reports, or the reports of trained
observers or expert judges is reduced. However, the potential for
confusing gender biases and real gender differences still exists. For
instance, a man who reports low anxiety in social situations during
the week may do so to conform with his perceptions of appropriate
male behavior. A woman may report many unpleasant reactions
from other people because she expects these and misinterprets feedback from others.

*Observation* either in simulated or real life contexts offers another
source of information. Criteria for judging effective behavior have
included the ratings of professionals based on interaction in simulated situations, peer ratings, reactions of significant others, and
the occurrence or non-occurrence of criterion behaviors, such as
refusing a request. Definitions of socially effective behavior differ
in the extent to which they consider both short term and long term
personal outcomes (effects on one's self) and social outcomes (effects on others). The opinions of experts and lay people may reflect
cultural stereotypes, and thus are not necessarily the best criterion to
use in assessing competence. Gender of the performer, of the judge
as well as characteristics of the situation influence evaluations that
are made. People expect men and women to use different power
bases (Johnson, 1976). Women speakers who use power bases
associated with another gender are liked less and regarded as less
competent and qualified than their male counterparts (Falbo, Hazen,
& Linimon, 1982). Activity on the part of women is often assessed
negatively (Costrich, Feinstein, Kedder, Maracek, & Pascale,
1975; Task Force on Sex Bias and Sex Role Stereotyping of the
American Psychological Association, 1975. See also Miller, 1974;
McDonald, 1982).

Kelly and others (1980) also found sex role bias in relation to female assertion. Subjects evaluated men and women responding assertively or unassertively to reasonable requests from strangers in public situations. Assertive women were evaluated as less competent, likable, and attractive than assertive males. Given the advantages and disadvantages of different sources of assessment information, it is best to use multiple sources including a balance of ''objective'' and ''subjective'' measures.

## Selecting Goals

Selection of goals is another important assessment task which can be influenced by gender of group leaders and group members. Biased observation may result in selection of goals that are not of maximal benefit or interest to the client. Decisions about the specific changes clients will strive to achieve may be biased by trainer and/ or client expectations of what are gender-appropriate goals for men and women (e.g., Broverman et al., 1975; Monahan, Kuhn, & Shaver, 1974). For example, reduction of anxiety in social situations may be viewed by the social worker as a more important goal for men compared to women since sex-role stereotypes define normal females as being more emotional and excitable (Broverman et al., 1975). A biased expectation of greater anxiety being ''normal'' among women is problematic in view of evidence that women who seek social skills training report high levels of anxiety (Hartsok, Olch, & deWolf, 1976; Brockway, 1976).

Assumptions may be inaccurate in terms of actual opportunities. What makes biased goal-setting by trainers especially troublesome is that the client may also accept dysfunctional sex-role stereotypes which unnecessarily limit options. If only the client holds such stereotypes, then an educational opportunity is at hand. The trainer can suggest or demonstrate to the client that options are broader than anticipated. Opportunities for education are especially rich in a group context. Group members who talk about their goals and expectations in specific social situations may offer models of gender-free or at least less stereotypic behaviors and options. If the group leader holds a dysfunctional stereotype not embraced by the client, then the client should seek professional help elsewhere. Acceptance of a stereotype by both the group worker and the group member is the most limiting combination since some options are completely hidden.

Failure to make distinctions among gender, gender identity,

gender role behaviors, and sexual orientation may result is inappropriate selection of goals and situations in which to pursue these. For example lesbian women may join a social skills group to increase contacts with other women, not with men, or their goals may be related to career advancement and not be relationship-focused. The sexual orientation of group members may not be at all obvious. This discretionary visibility (whether sexual orientation is disclosed) may mislead a trainer into making faulty assumptions about desired goals. Reluctance to disclose a deviant sexual orientation may be increased by failure of the trainer to overtly recognize alternative life style.

Part of being sensitive to gender differences in social skills training, is being knowledgeable about rules related to social situations of concern to clients and gender differences that pertain to these. Although achieving equality of opportunities in all situations may be an optimal goal to pursue in the long run, in terms of current goals of individual clients, these may only be partially attainable because of societal values and norms. It is the social skills trainer who should be knowledgeable about the probability of a particular goal being successfully pursued in a specific situation by a woman or a man. For example, a woman might like to increase her social contacts and to become more active in asking men (or women) out. The trainer is responsible for identifying situations in which the client is likely to be effective (positively received) and those in which she is not likely to succeed (be rejected). It is not enough for the trainer to say that certain goals cannot be pursued. The trainer must offer more than this. Cognitive restructuring may be required in which the value of goals is reassessed. Or, other procedures for attaining goals which will be more effective than social skills or assertion training can be suggested such as the formation of support groups among women, one purpose of which is to take action as a group in order to achieve a certain goal, such as a decrease in gender bias among judges. It is also the trainer's responsibility to help the client, perhaps with the assistance of other group members, to explore possible advantages and disadvantages of achieving specific goals. Only in this way is the client in an informed position to conduct a cost-benefit analysis in relation to pursuing specific outcomes. Helping clients make decisions about various goal options may be facilitated by having members complete a Decision-Making Worksheet (Morton, Richey, & Kellett, 1981). This worksheet provides step-by-step guidelines for selecting the option which has the greatest probability of positive consequences in a particular situation.

## Selecting Progress Indicators

Clients have a right to know whether they are achieving their goals or not. This right can be truly offered if goals are clear and progress indicators are selected by the client. Allowing the client to select progress indicators will eliminate many sources of potential gender bias. Progress indicators should be selected at an early point and monitored throughout the training program so that both the trainer and the client can determine the degree of progress and take appropriate next steps in accord with what is found. Tools used to gather assessment information, can be used to assess progress during training. Obtaining feedback on client satisfaction with treatment is important but does not substitute for on-going feedback concerning goal attainment. Relying on client satisfaction introduces potential gender bias in determining effectiveness, especially if the clients are women. Because of their socialization, women may be especially prone to offer positive feedback despite lack of goal attainment because they do not wish to offend the leader by being critical. The extent to which a program allows participants to achieve specific goals should be the principle criterion used to determine program effectiveness. Other writers who have discussed gender and the use of behavioral methods have also stressed this measure of effectiveness (e.g., Blechman, 1980).

## Selection of Intervention Focus

It is via assessment that the trainer identifies not only *what* goals the client desires, but how these can best be pursued. Should the client change how he responds in real life settings, how he thinks about events, or, should aspects of the environment be changed? Gender biases have been found in relation to selection of factors related to presenting problems. For example, Bowman (1982) found that therapists are more likely to attribute relationship discord to intrapsychic problems in women which require insight treatment, whereas the same problem among men was viewed as an interpersonal relationship problem requiring couples therapy.

## INTERVENTION CONSIDERATIONS

Social skills training consists of a variety of components, including model presentation, behavior rehearsal or role playing, feedback, coaching or guidance, social and self-reinforcement, and homework assignments. The nature of each person's goals and related cognitive, physiological and behavioral asets, deficits and surfeits should be considered in the design of procedures as well as group process variables. As in assessment, gender biases and ignorance of gender differences can influence the selection of procedures.

Social skills trainers must decide whether social skills or assertion training is the procedure of choice to help clients reach their goals. It may not be, or, it may comprise only one aspect of intervention. Inequities of power distribution will usually not be altered by helping clients learn more effective social skills. Effective social skills may help to decrease such differences in some situations but these will not make such differences disappear. In such situations, clients may benefit more from acquiring skills in other areas such as knowledge about organizational sources of power and clear thinking skills which will be of help in identifying and countering faulty arguments. Social skills training may focus on helping women to develop support systems and groups that can be used to pursue goals desired by group members.

## Offering Training in Component Skills

Social skills trainers must decide what specific verbal and nonverbal behaviors to increase, decrease, vary or stabilize in order to aid clients in attaining desired goals. This will require knowledge about the likely outcomes of specific behaviors in specific situations for both men and women. Ignorance about gender differences on the part of the trainer will be very problematic. This may result in training clients in ineffective behaviors. Inappropriate models may be presented and incorrect verbal and nonverbal skills may be selected to focus on during rehearsal and feedback. Errors of omission may be made as well as errors of commission; it is just as important to know when not to engage in a behavior as when to perform it in order to be socially effective.

For example, what particular behaviors are associated with being a valuable participant (or leader) in a group discussion or meeting? Are their "core" or generic behaviors that are associated with effective interaction and leadership for both men and women, such as eye contact with other group members, adequate voice volume, and elaboration on comments? Particular behaviors may have to be changed to overcome limitations imposed by sex-role socialization.

Women may require additional training in expressing and defending their opinions, resisting interruption, and talking for longer periods of time (Hall, 1978). Men may require additional training in attending and listening skills (Davis & Weitz, 1981; Zimmerman & West, 1975), and in interpreting nonverbal messages from others (Frieze et al., 1978; Hall, 1978).

Behaviors that are viewed as inappropriate for the gender of the person will often result in negative consequences from others. Both men and women negatively evaluate women who use nonverbal behaviors that are considered gender-inappropriate (Mehrabian, 1972). Speakers using expressions of power associated with another gender are liked less and regarded as less competent and qualified than their counterparts (Falbo, Hazen, & Linimon, 1982). It is important that social workers be knowledgeable about sources of power in different situations and help to educate their clients about these (Smith & Grenier, 1982; Kanter, 1979).

## Selecting Homework Assignments

Attention to inappropriate behavioral components will decrease the likelihood that clients will experience success when carrying out homework assignments in real-life settings. Ignorance about the ways in which gender differences influence what goals can be successfully pursued in specific situations for men and for women will compound the negative effects of training clients in effective verbal and non-verbal skills.

Trainers should assist clients to develop responses which are likely to increase positive outcomes while also decreasing the likelihood of negative reactions. This will require knowledge about gender differences and sex role stereotypes. The amount and timing of gender-related behaviors is as important in relation to social competence as their occurrence or nonoccurrence. A trainer might advise a woman not to smile during group meetings at work since smiling is associated with a submissiveness and lower status and will decrease her credibility and influence (Frieze & Ramsey, 1976). If this advice were followed, the outcome might be more negative than positive, especially if this woman has used smiling in the past to facilitate her interactions. She could be advised instead to reduce but not to eliminate verbal and nonverbal expressions of warmth (e.g., smiling), or to express warmth and liking at times which *reinforce others* for attending to and considering *her* contributions. An empathic-assertive response, which combines verbal and nonverbal assertive components and expressions of understanding and concern, may result in favorable consequences (Kern, 1982).

Failure to recognize the relationship between gender and status differences may result in incorrect advice to clients. For example, a woman who wishes to assume a greater leadership role where she works might be advised to sit at the head of the table during staff meetings. This might be risky advice since Porter and Geis (1981) have shown that assuming a high status position in a group may not be effective for a woman. Advice to use more direct power signals would also be poor since women's use of stronger, more direct power signals is likely to incur rejection (Frieze, 1978). What should a trainer suggest?

What options are available? Social consensus among group members concerning a woman's leadership role (Brown, 1980) and increasing social support by making sure the group includes a same-sex peer (Porter, 1980) have been found to be helpful. Another possibility is encouraging clients to first use the "minimal effective response" in a situation (Rimm & Masters, 1974). This response includes behaviors that are likely to result in goal accomplishment with minimal effort and a low probability of adverse consequences. If a woman wants to increase her influence as a public speaker, she should begin practicing with topics that are viewed as gender-appropriate (Falbo, Hazen, & Linimon, 1982). Clients should learn to make small changes in their own behavior including reinforcing others for changes in their reactions. Other options include forming social support groups and helping clients to develop their skills in other areas that may not involve social skills.

Clients should be prepared for possible adverse consequences resulting from new behaviors. Both overt and covert coping responses can be developed, modeled, and rehearsed in group sessions before clients carry out potentially risky assignments in real-life.

### Attending to Cognitive and Emotional Variables

Time may have to be devoted to the exploration of dysfunctional beliefs about sex roles and options for change. Gender biases and ignorance about gender differences may impede recognition of important cognitive and emotional reactions that influence social competence. For example, a trainer may assume that men do not worry about rejection as much as women in social situations so fail to include procedures to decrease male clients' dysfunctional thoughts and increase helpful ones. Or, a trainer may not attend to or explore the feelings of men as readily as she or he attends to the feelings of women (Marecek & Johnson, 1980). Problems may also arise because trainers view women's anticipation of negative consequences for increased assertion as largely resulting from irrational beliefs or erroneous expectations (Linehan & Egan, 1979), and overlook negative sanctions that may follow gender-inappropriate behavior. Certainly, fear of performing a particular behavior may be due to unfounded expectations of social punishment. A recent study of male undergraduate students found that if a man liked a woman, she could ask him out for a date without fear of negative consequences for taking the initiative (Muehlenhard & McFall, 1981). However, as these authors and others (e.g., Linehan & Egan, 1979) have pointed out, self-reports may differ from actual responses to assertive women. A stereotype that women are more emotional than men may result in failure to offer women clients appropriate stress-management skills that will facilitate effective social behavior.

## SUMMARY

Social skills training is used with children, youth and adults to enhance interpersonal competencies. Specific intervention components should be selected based on an individualized assessment. Gender stereotypes, confusions among gender, role behaviors, gender identity, and sexual orientation, and ignorance concerning gender differences related to effective behavior in specific situations, may intrude during assessment as well as during intervention and decrease the quality of training offered to clients. These may result in restricting options considered, selection of an inappropriate focus of intervention (for example, attending to individual pathology rather than environmental constraints), and incorrect selection of component skills. A focus on both personal and social outcomes achieved as a measure of progress rather than component skills will be helpful in decreasing intrusion of sex role stereotypes. The unconscious nature of stereotypes calls for vigilence to insure that biased views do not unduly influence selection of outcomes and ways to achieve these.

64      GROUPWORK WITH WOMEN/GROUPWORK WITH MEN

# REFERENCES

Alberti, R. E. and Emmons, M. L. *Your perfect right.* San Luis Obispo, Calif.: *Impact* (2nd Ed.), 1982.

Alden, L., and Cappe, R. Nonassertiveness: Skill deficit or selective self-evaluation? *Behavior Therapy,* 1981, *12,* 107-114.

American Psychological Association Report of the Task Force on Sex Bias and Sex-Role Stereotyping in Psychotherapeutic Practice. *American Psychologist,* 1975, *30,* 1169-1175.

Argyle, M., Furnham, A., and Graham, J. A. *Social situations.* Cambridge: Cambridge Univ. Press, 1981.

Blechman, E. A. Behavior therapies. In A. M. Brodsky and R. T. Hare-Mustin (Eds.), *Women and psychotherapy: An assessment of research and practice.* New York: Guilford Press, 1980, 217-244.

Brockway, B. S. Assertive training for professional women. *Social Work,* 1976, *21,* 498-505.

Broverman, I. K., Voegel, S. R., Broverman, D. M., Clarkson, F. E., and Rosen-Krantz, P. S. Sex-role stereotypes: A current appraisal. In M. Mednick, S. Tangri, and L. Hoffman (Eds.), *Women and achievement.* New York: John Wiley & Sons, 1975.

Brown, V. Illegitimate context influence on evaluation of male and female leadership performance. Unpub. doc. disser. University of Delaware, 1980.

Campbell, D. T. Stereotypes and the perception of group differences. *American Psychologist,* 1967, *22,* 817-829.

Costrich, N., Feinstein, J., Kedder, L., Marecek, J., and Pascale, L. When stereotypes hurt: Three studies of penalties for sex role reversals. *Journal of Experimental Social Psychology,* 1975, *11,* 520-530.

Crosby, F., Jose, P., and Wong-McCarthy, W. Gender, androgyny, and conversational assertiveness. In C. Mayo and N. M. Henley (Eds.), *Gender and nonverbal behavior.* New York: Springer-Verlag, 1981.

Davis, M. and Weitz, S. Sex differences in body movements and positions. In C. Mayo and N. M. Henley (Eds.), *Gender and nonverbal behavior.* New York: Springer-Verlag, 1981.

Eisler, R. M., Frederiksen, L. W., and Peterson, G. L. The relationship of cognitive variables to the expression of assertiveness. *Behavior Therapy,* 1978, *9,* 419-427.

Falbo, T., Hazen, M. D., and Linimon, D. The costs of selecting power bases or messages associated with the opposite sex. *Sex Roles,* 1982, *8,* 147-157.

Frieze, I. H. Being feminine or masculine nonverbally. In I. H. Frieze, J. E. Parsons, P. B. Johnson, N. Ruble, and G. L. Zellman (Eds.), *Women and sex roles: A social psychological perspective.* New York: Norton, 1978.

Frieze, I. H. and Ramsey, S. J. Nonverbal maintenance of traditional sex-roles. *Journal of Social Issues,* 1976, *32,* 133-141.

Furnham, A. and Argyle, M. The theory, practice and application of social skills training. *Interpersonal Journal of Behavioural Social Work and Abstracts,* 1981, *1,* 215-144.

Gambrill, E. D. *Behavior modification: Handbook of assessment, intervention and evaluation.* San Francisco: Jossey-Bass, 1977.

Gambrill, E. D. and Richey, C. A. An assertion inventory for use in assessment and research. *Behavior Therapy,* 1975, *6,* 547-549.

Gambrill, E. D. and Richey, C. A. *Shy or sociable: It's up to you,* (2nd Ed.). New York: Harper and Row, in press.

Glass, C. R. and Merluzzi, T. V. Cognitive assessment of social-evaluative anxiety. In T. V. Merluzzi, C. R. Glass, and M. Genest (Eds.), *Cognitive assessment.* New York: Guilford Press, 1981, 388-438.

Grady, K. E. Sex bias in research design. *Psychology of Women Quarterly,* 1981, *5,* 628-636.

Hall, J. A. Gender effects in decoding nonverbal cues. *Psychological Bulletin,* 1978, *85,* 845-857.

Harré, R. and Secord, P. *The explanation of social behavior.* Oxford: Blackwell, 1972.

Hartsook, J. E., Olch, D. R., and deWolf, V. A. Personality characteristics of women's assertiveness training group participants. *Journal of Counseling Psychology,* 1976, *23,* 322-326.

Jakubowski, P. and Lange, A. J. *The assertive option: Your rights and responsibilities.* Champaign, Ill.: Research Press, 1978.

Johnson, P. B. Women and power: Toward a theory of effectiveness. *Journal of Social Issues,* 1976, *32,* 99-110.

Kanter, R. Differential access to opportunity and power. In R. Alvarez, K. G. Lutterman, and Associates. *Discrimination in organizations.* San Francisco: Jossey-Bass, 1979.

Kelly, J. A., Kern, J. M., Kirkley, B. G., Patterson, J. N., and Keane, T. M. Reactions to assertive versus unassertive behavior: Differential effects for males and females and implications for assertive training. *Behavior Therapy,* 1980, *11,* 670-682.

Kern, J. M. Predicting the impact of assertive, empathic-assertive, and non-assertive behavior: The assertiveness of the assertee. *Behavior Therapy,* 1982, *13,* 486-498.

Kiecolt, J., and McGrath, E. Social desirability responding in the measurement of assertive behavior. *Journal of Consulting and Clinical Psychology,* 1979, *47,* 640-642.

Linehan, M. M., and Egan, K. J. Assertion training for women. In A. S. Bellack and M. Hersen (Eds.), *Research and practice in social skills training.* New York: Plenum, 1979.

Mayo, C. and Henley, N. M. (Eds.), *Gender and nonverbal behavior.* New York: Springer-Verlag, 1981.

MacDonald, M. L. Assertion training for women. In J. P. Curran and P. M. Monti (Eds.), *Social skills training: A practical handbook for assessment and treatment.* New York: The Guilford Press, 1982.

Marecek, J., and Johnson, M. Gender and the process of therapy. In A. M. Brodsky and R. Hare-Mustin (Eds.), *Women and psychotherapy: An assessment of research and practice.* New York: The Guilford Press, 1980.

McFall, R. M. A review and reformulation of the concept of social skills. *Behavioral Assessment,* 1982, *4,* 1-33.

Mehrabian, A. Nonverbal communication. Chicago: Aldine Atherton, 1972.

Miller, D. The influence of the patient's sex on clinical judgement. *Smith College Studies in Social Work,* 1974, *44,* 89-100.

Mischel, W. A cognitive-social learning approach to assessment. In T. V. Merluzzi, C. R. Glass, and M. Genest (Eds.), *Cognitive assessment.* New York: Guilford Press, 1981.

Monahan, L., Kuhn, D., and Shaver, P. Intrapsychic versus cultural explanations of the 'fear of success' motive. *Journal of Personality and Social Psychology,* 1974, *29,* 60-64.

Morrison, R. L., and Bellack, A. S. The role of social perception in social skill. *Behavior Therapy,* 1981, *12,* 69-79.

Morton, J. C., Richey, C. A., and Kellett, M. *Building assertive skills: A practical guide to professional development for allied dental health providers.* St. Louis: The C. V. Mosby Company, 1981.

Muehlenhard, C. L., and McFall, R. M. Dating initiation from a woman's perspective. *Behavior Therapy,* 1981, *12,* 682-691.

Porter, N. and Geis, F. Women and nonverbal leadership cues: When seeing is not believing. In C. Mayo and N. M. Henley (Eds.), *Gender and Nonverbal Behavior.* New York: Springer-Verlag, 1981.

Rimm, D. C., and Masters, J. C. *Behavior therapy: Techniques and empirical findings.* New York: Academic Press, 1974.

Sherman, J., Koufacos, C., and Kenworthy, J. A. Therapists: Their attitudes and information about women. *Psychology of Women Quarterly,* 1978, *2,* 299-313.

Smith, H. L., and Grenier, M. Sources of organizational power for women: Overcoming structural obstacles. *Sex Roles,* 1982, *8,* 733-746.

Thorne, B. and Henley, N. (Eds.), *Language and sex: Difference and dominance.* Rowley, MA: Newbury House, 1975.

Thouless, R. H. *Straight and crooked thinking.* London: Pan Books, 1974.

Trower, P. Toward a generative model of social skills: A critique and synthesis. In J. P.

Curran and P. M. Monti (Eds.), *Social skills training.* New York: The Guilford Press, 1982.

Zimmerman, D. H. and West, C. Sex roles, interruptions, and silences in conversation. In B. Thorne and N. Henley (Eds.), *Language and sex: Differences and dominance.* Rowley, MA: Newbury House, 1975.

# Sexual Identity Issues in Group Work: Gender, Social Sex Role, and Sexual Orientation Considerations

Tom Morson
Robert McInnis

**ABSTRACT.** Polarized thinking about gender, social sex roles, and sexual orientation has resulted in sexual identity confusion. In this article group interventions for work with this confusion will be presented. Confounding as it relates to issues involved in the development of homosexual identities will be described, as will "coming out" groups as interventions for homosexual exploration. Finally, a screening procedure for sexual identity confusion groups will be presented.

Strong cultural prescriptions about how men and women should be "masculine" or "feminine"—in work, mannerisms, physical attributes, interests, sexual desire, thoughts, feelings, and behaviors—has led to polarized thinking about sexual identity. Individuals are perceived as either masculine or feminine, heterosexual or homosexual. This either/or thinking has contributed to the fear that is at the root of much sexism and, in particular, homo/heterophobia. A number of researchers, theorists, and practitioners (Shively & DeCecco, 1977; Solomon, 1982; Sherif, 1982) have urged that we make more distinctions among the various component parts of sexual identity.

In this paper, we will first outline these components and discuss the ways they are often confounded in the understanding of sexual

Tom Morson is Senior Counselor, Counseling Services, University of Michigan, Ann Arbor, 3100 Michigan Union Building, Ann Arbor, MI 48109. Robert McInnis is an intern at Counseling Services, University of Michigan, 1982-1983.

*67*

identity. We will then briefly describe this confounding as it relates to issues involved in the development of homosexual identities. Finally, we will describe some group interventions for work with sexual identity confusion particularly as it relates to issues of gender and sex roles.

Exploration of the ways in which the various aspects of sexual identity are often confused is likely to be important for anyone interested in examining their self-concept, behavior, and relationships, and will be especially important in all-men's, all-women's, or mixed groups formed explicitly to explore issues related to gender roles and socialization.

## COMPONENTS OF SEXUAL IDENTITY

As noted in Garvin and Reed (this volume), Shively and DeCecco (1977) define four separate but interlinked concepts as components of sexual identity: (1) biological sex; (2) gender identity; (3) social sex role, and (4) sexual orientation.

> Biological Sex: male and female are usually readily identifiable by external sex organs, or by hormonal levels and chromosomal structure.

> Gender Identity: the individual's basic conviction of being male or female (develops between birth and three years of age and is part of the internalized cognitive and affective self-identification).

> Social Sex Role: behaviors and characteristics, defined by self and reinforced by others as the ways "boys/men or girls/women" behave (thought to develop between ages three to seven).

> Sexual Orientation: refers to affectional/cognitive and physical *preference* for a partner (parallels but is not synchronous with development of social sex roles).

These components are frequently confused with sexual identity concerns. Conflicts of biological sex and gender identity (transexualism) and gender identity and social sex role (transvestism) are, for example, often regarded as degrees of homosexuality. Perhaps more insidious is the confounding of conflicts between social sex role and sexual orientation which often results in a client being mislabeled by self or others as a homosexual. Education about these terms and the differences among them is essential if people are to untangle the ways these issues are intertwined for them.

Unfortunately, the common tendency is not to differentiate, but rather to label a variety of behaviors, cognitions, and affects as homosexual. This mislabeling may extend to the lack of sexual desire (asexuality), dysfunctional heterosexuality, and bisexuality), dysfunctional heterosexuality, and bisexuality. This mislabeling, we believe, is fueled by homophobia (fear of the homosexual) and the resulting widespread simplistic and polarized thinking about masculinity and femininity and heterosexuality and homosexuality. Rigid bipolar thinking about identity in general does not do justice to the complexity of the human condition. This kind of thinking also contributes to the splitting off of the affective and cognitive from the behavioral. For those in the throes of either a homosexual, heterosexual, or bisexual orientation identity conflict, the lack of positive sanctioning in the culture of multiplistic modes of being contributes to the inability to accept ones own feelings, thoughts and behaviors as "normal."

Social workers must be prepared to deal with confusion among these concepts as it is likely to arise in many types of groups. In fact, it may be unclear for some time with some people whether they really are experiencing a homosexual, heterosexual, bisexual, gender, or sex role concern. Homo/heterophobia results in these issues being labeled as homosexual.

Several authors have outlined stage models of homosexual identity/orientation development [Cass (1979), Troiden (1979), and Coleman (1982)]. Gonsiorek (1982) offers an excellent review of the many difficulties in assessment, particularly when homosexual concerns are presented with longstanding character problems.

These authors are concerned with the processes by which one identifies aspects of self or self as homosexual and stress: (1) that a homosexual orientation is self-determined; (2) involves affective, cognitive, and behavioral preferences; (3) frequently involves processes characterized by confusion; fear of rejection and ambivalence; and (4) the need for more research on homosexual identity formation.

Frequently one in the throes of developing a homosexual identity is struggling with gender and sex role issues. It is our contention that unconditional support for the exploration of the confusion is critical.

Further, it has been our experience that groups led by leaders' accepting and facilitating of multiplistic modes of being best allow individuals to determine for themselves their preferences.

## SEXUAL IDENTITY CONFUSION IN GROUP

I've decided I must be gay since I'm not like other men; I like cooking and housework. I don't know what to do about it. I'm feeling panicky. I thought by this age it would have worked itself out.

The labeling of some dimension/aspect of self as different, and then as homosexual, in this example is representative of conflicts between perceived sex role expectation fulfillment, gender identity and sexual orientation. Because he enjoys tasks that are socially defined as feminine (social sex role), he calls into question some sense of his basic conviction of maleness (gender identity), which then raises questions regarding his basic sexual orientation. To enjoy tasks that are feminine is understood as not being masculine and then further as homosexual.

He may or may not be in the initial stages of developing a homosexual identity. He most definitely is in some distress and is labeling behaviors as homosexual that, in fact, have nothing to do with homosexuality.

This concern was initially presented to one of the authors during a routine initial screening appointment at the University of Michigan Counseling Services. Since a group was available that had as its focus sexual identity and larger relationship issues and since the group was being co-led by one of the authors, it was decided to place him in the group.

This group consisted of 7 members, 3 men, 4 women. Members were screened by both the male and female leaders and were told that the group would be using videotape. All of the individuals were concerned with sexuality; and none were currently in any kind of significant intimate personal relationship. Four (2 of the women and 2 of the men) were concerned about sexual orientation.

The client in question was one of these. He was very verbal, athletic, and attractive in appearance. John (pseudonym) was the youngest and only male in a family of 4 sibs. His parents had been divorced since he was 5. He seldom if ever saw his father who had moved to the opposite coast and remarried. John reported that as the only male in his family he felt a great deal of pressure to help keep the family together. Although his stature, mannerisms, and general way of presenting himself appeared to conform to general male stereotypes, John's internal sense of his "appropriateness" was lacking. He reported feeling very anxious and fearful when in groups of all men as well as having thoughts of not being as capable, aggressive, and attracted to women as other men. He reported attraction for both men and women but no strong physical attractions for either.

Based on this information, our tentative assessment was that John was in the throes of gender identity and sex role confusion. Like others we had worked with, there had been a strong lack of male models throughout early socialization, as well as a sense of desire for male affiliation with no clearly reported sense of physical desire for either sex. We wondered if John's interests in housework and cooking were not his ways of assuming a sense of familial expectation and his way of keeping the family together. As the youngest, John caused us to wonder about his struggles to leave his family and, in particular, about his conflicts with his mother and sisters who, like him, felt an acute desire for male parental guidance.

Like others experiencing confusion in this group, John had tremendous splits among his behaviors, affects and cognitions. What follows is a description of some of the techniques that were employed in working with the confusion, confounding, and polarization that these members were experiencing.

### Reframing and Educating

Reframing the confusion as normal and facilitating exploration of it in all its many aspects is critical. This can best be done by education as to the behavioral, cognitive, and affective aspects of the identity confusion, followed by focusing on the stress experienced in each. We employ part of the two hour group time for education on specific topics since the confusion often results from lack of information and polarized thinking and feelings. The remaining time is used for personal work related to each of the topics presented. In the group under discussion, the topics presented were: family—the first socialization experience; identity development—with a particular focus on sexual identity development; stress as a reaction to lack of congruence between sexuality and sex roles; and masculinity and femininity.

## Family—The First Socialization Experience

In this presentation we stress that the family is the first group in which we are socialized and that, as such, we first learn the basics about self and self in relationship to the world. We asked participants to bring family pictures and to spend time exploring the many messages and roles learned in the family. In John's case, for example, he was able to gain understanding that his interests were not related to his sense of self but rather to what his family expected of him and his response to this expectation. John also was able to begin to discuss his lack of male models and his desire to have more male affiliation. Other members solicited his feelings and gave support by sharing their feelings about their abilities and inabilities to meet family expectations.

## Identity-Sexual Identity

Here we present the model as outlined by DeCecco and Shively (1977) and spend time explaining each component part. During this discussion, John became acutely aware that his concerns seemed to be more related to gender and sex role than one of sexual preference.

## Stress—Thinking, Feeling, Behaving

We normalize stress as a reaction to our environment, our thoughts, feelings and behaviors. We teach the differences between each and how this can be experienced so as to result in lowered self-esteem and approach-avoidance conflicts. In this group we used an exercise in which we had each member write five thoughts, feelings, and behaviors that they labeled as masculine and feminine and then used this lead to our discussion of masculinity and femininity. John became more aware of how his absence of male models had resulted in stress that then affected his thinking, feelings, and behavior in terms of comfort with his masculinity. Group members supported him and shared their own difficulties with stress related to their sense of sexual identity. John began to actively mourn the loss of a father and acknowledged that he felt that he was inferior because of this.

## Masculinity/Femininity

Here, we used their own labeling based on the above exercise and focused particularly on cultural assumptions and rigidity about "shoulds" in this area. We stressed the concept of androgyny and asked each to identify the positive masculine and feminine aspects of themselves. John, for example, learned that his cooking and housework interests were really survival skills and strengths. For homework we asked each to go into a card shop and pick out two male and two female birth announcements and bring them to the next group for discussion. We then analyzed them with a focus on the many symbols, colors, words, attitudes, that were being used to represent masculine/feminine.

## Sexuality/Sex Roles

Here we put up newsprint on the walls with the following words: male, female, man, woman, boy, girl, masculine, feminine, lady, gentleman, heterosexual, sexual, homosexual, bisexual on the top. We then asked that members spend the next 20 minutes in silence moving to each sheet and writing their first association. As leaders, we too participated and when necesary wrote down slang words to facilitate further disclosure. We then asked each member to pick two sheets, and to read aloud each of the words after telling why they chose the sheet they chose.

John chose "homosexual" and "feminine" and reported that he picked these sheets because these were two words that evoked strong responses in him.

We have found this exercise helpful in bringing out strong negative self labeling and in evoking discussion of this labeling and its impact on sexual identity development.

## Use of Videotape

We videotaped the second and fourth sessions of this 18 session, 2 hour weekly group. We then played back still shots of each person and had each give feedback as to what they were seeing and feeling. Videotape feedback facilitates cohesion and allows for body image distortion correction which seems to be frequently reported by those experiencing confusion. We focus first on the individual giving feedback to the video-image of self and then open it to the group for their feedback. John learned that he, in fact, does present well and this was confirmed by other members' feedback.

In the course of this group experience John became increasingly more assertive, relaxed and self disclosing. He contracted with the group to ask out a young woman in one of his classes, which he, in fact, did. He seemed less concerned with whether or not he was gay/homosexual and more self accepting. At last report John was dating a woman he had met at church.

Other members went through similar experiences. Two of the members (one not originally expressing sexual orientation concerns) began to allow these feelings to emerge. One of these contracted with the group to attend a local Gay Liberation Front Meeting and to report on his experience. At this meeting he learned of a "coming out" group that was forming and eventually he decided to join. The group was supportive of his exploration efforts and encouraged him to share his impressions with other members. He stated that he had heard of such groups before but was too afraid to attend. He now felt more comfortable exploring his same-sex feelings with the knowledge that he had group support.

## COMING OUT GROUPS

As this client began to explore these feelings, he had a desire to test and compare his experiences with others. For this reason, a "coming-out" group composed of others experiencing similar feelings, thoughts and behaviors seems to be most beneficial. We realize that frequently such groups are not available as interventions and thus recommend that the worker think about contacting local homosexual/gay organizations or hotlines for assistance.

"Coming-out" groups are groups composed of same sex individuals who have identified some aspect of self (affect, cognition, behavior) as homosexual and wish to explore the implications of this identification further. This identification results tentatively in the adoption of the gay/homosexual orientation sexual identity. The purposes of coming-out groups are (1) to introduce the client to the local gay community and its norms; (2) to allow for continued support, exploration, and ventilation of concerns; (3) to reduce a sense of alienation/anomie; and (4) to educate the individual regarding gay/lesbian sexuality and community resources, these goals are achieved by providing opportunities to compare and contrast experiences with others, and multiple models of coping style, attitudes, and behavior.

Most of these groups are offered by, or in conjunction with, gay community center personnel, and are frequently peer led. Gay-identified workers can employ the use of appropriate self-disclosure to facilitate this process.

Where gender or sex role is the primary concern or confusion is too great, we feel a "coming out" group is contraindicated because the client may:

1. *not* be "coming out" to a homosexual orientation;
2. need careful attention in an open ended group or individual counseling situation to assist with confounding, self negation, polarization, etc.; or
3. be highly susceptible to peer pressure.

Where concerns center on gender or sex roles, and the individual does not seem to be dealing with sexual orientation concerns, men's or women's groups are highly recommended. For more information on these groups see the other articles in this issue.

### Sexual Identity Confusion: Other Considerations for Group Work

*Screening.* Referral and placement in a group of those experiencing sexual identity confusion is frequently met with resistance, fear, and anxiety on the part of the client. Often these concerns are experienced as unique and there is a tremendous amount of shame and guilt associated with disclosing them to others. For this reason we strongly recommend screening focused on: (1) education as to the nature, importance, and focus of the group; (2) assessment of the degree of anxiety and ability to give and receive feedback in a group setting; and (3) developing initial rapport that will help to allay the anxiety.

We routinely share with members that it is natural to feel anxious and uncertain and that others will be in the group who are experiencing similar concerns. We inform them that we are planning a small group experience (6-8 members), how long we plan to meet, the time, the place, and the format. We stress confidentiality. We ask that they make a commitment to attend the first three sessions.

Then, should they want to drop out they may, but we ask them to discuss their reasons with us and the group. We encourage them to ask any questions they might have about us or the group. We also share our initial impressions and reactions of them and ask that they do so as well. We allot approximately one-half hour for this screening appointment. We screen out those who seem to be too crisis or anxiety ridden to tolerate a group, use this time to begin framing their concern in a social context and to prepare them for the experience. We strongly recommend that for groups focused on sexual identity concerns the leaders, and not the intake worker do the screening.

*Membership.* We recommend that there be a mixed membership with contrasting gender, sex role and sexual orientation concerns. In our experience this variety offers many models of attitudes, styles of coping, and behaviors. We have led same-sex groups with a variety of sexual identity concerns and found that they were useful, but as one member put it in his evaluation, "he wanted to see how the other sex would react."

## CONCLUDING REMARKS

There is a pressing need for research in the processes that facilitate the exploration of sexual identity concerns, the development of healthy homosexual orientations, and the kinds of group services that best facilitate these. Thorough assessment and sensitivity to the components of sexual identity is needed. Clients are likely to continue to have difficulties in these areas given the tremendous oppression, polarization and confounding that exists in the culture.

Groups designed with these components seem to assist with the clearing of confusion and allow for the necessary exploration to achieve a fuller sense of sexual identity. We have described one such group in the hopes that it will prompt others leading such groups to report their experiences in the group work literature.

### REFERENCES

Cass, V. C. Homosexual identity formation: A theoretical model. *Journal of Homosexuality,* 1979, *4,* 219-235.

Coleman, E. Developmental stages in the coming out process. Homosexuality and psychotherapy: A practitioner's handbook of affirmative models. *Journal of Homosexuality,* 1982, *7*(2/3), 31-43.

Gonsiorek, J. The use of diagnostic concepts in working with gay and lesbian populations. Homosexuality and psychotherapy: A practitioner's handbook of affirmative models. *Journal of Homosexuality,* 1982, *7*(2/3), 9-19.

Sherif, C. W. Needed concepts in the study of gender identity. *Psychology of Women Quarterly,* 1982, *6,* 375-398.

Shively, M. G. and DeCecco, J. P. Components of sexual identity. *Journal of Homosexuality,* 1977, *3*(1), 41-48.

Solomon, K. The masculine gender role: Description. In K. Solomon and N. B. Levy (eds.), *Men in Transition: Changing Male Roles, Theory and Therapy.* New York: Plenum Press, 1983.

Troiden, R. R. Becoming homosexual: A model of gay identity acquisition. *Psychiatry,* 1979, *42*(Nov.).

Yalom, I. *The Theory and Practice of Group Psychotherapy* (2nd Edition). New York: Basic Books, 1975.

# PRACTICE WITH WOMEN

# The Distinctive Attributes
# of Feminist Groups

Naomi Gottlieb
Dianne Burden
Ruth McCormick
Ginny Nicarthy

**ABSTRACT.** Using the experience of four groups—single parent, abused women, women returning to school, and assertive skills trainees—the paper makes the central point that feminist oriented groups create special circumstances to counteract harmful sex-role socialization. These special factors include: (1) a decrease in women's particular isolation from each other, (2) an emphasis on social and political factors in women's lives, (3) the absence of men in the group, (4) the development in women of group facilitation skills. In light of the effects of these distinctive aspects, the authors suggest that facilitators of groups with female participants consider whether their approach meets women's special needs sufficiently.

Facilitators of all-female feminist groups have been aware for some time of a number of factors which appear unique to different types of feminist groups as well as common to all of them, whatever their specific purpose. This article attempts to systematize both the uniqueness and the commonalities of such groups. It draws on the experience of four types of groups and makes the central point that feminist-oriented groups create special circumstances for women participants which are intended to counteract some of the harmful effects of sex-role socialization. The primary factors contributing to this impact include: (1) the particular nature of the decrease in

Naomi Gottlieb is Professor, School of Social Work, University of Washington, 4101-15th Avenue NE, Seattle, WA 98195. Dianne Burden is Assistant Professor, School of Social Work, Boston University, 755 Commonwealth Avenue, Boston, MA 02215. Ruth McCormick is Director, Women's Studies Program, Edmonds Community College, Lynnwood, WA 98036. Ginny Nicarthy is with Women's Counseling Group, 2800 East Madison, Seattle, WA 98112, and is founder and former director of Abused Women's Network, Women's Institute, Seattle, Washington.

women's isolation from one another, (2) an emphasis on the social and political factors in women's lives, (3) the absence of men in the groups, and (4) the development of leadership skills among the women themselves. The four groups utilized in the discussion—single parents, abused women, mature women returning to school, and assertive skills trainees—provide examples of these common features. Although there are variations in the groups, the similarities are striking. Whatever the rationale for the group, the leaders, using a feminist perspective, provide women with an awareness of the impact of women's place in a sexist society, and facilitate the development of skills to counteract the negative impact of socialization.

The discussion is not a report of an empirical study of these factors, though the material is partly based on participants' responses in regularly administered systematic evaluations at the close of some of the groups. Careful and systematic investigations of the prevalence and effects of the group processes discussed here are needed and would add greatly to the literature. Prior to such systematic study, however, a report of group facilitators' experiences appear warranted since the common features of feminist groups are becoming more and more evident.

## Description of the Groups

The four groups vary considerably in their central purpose and format. The *groups for abused women* are intended for women caught in or recovering from relationships with men who batter. The women attend weekly drop-in sessions, some coming for many months, others just a few times. It is important that new members have ready access to the group at a time when they are prepared to consider changes and that they have the opportunity to meet in a group with women who have already taken some of the steps they are considering.

The *classes for returning women* are part of the regular curriculum at a community college and the goal is to provide an atmosphere in which women can gain enough self-confidence, assertiveness, and social skills to enter the mainstream of the college and become successful students, or to enter the labor market and obtain jobs. The unique feature of the program is the "home base" or women's class, with its consciousness-raising component, taken concurrently with remedial and developmental classes, such as reading improvement, basic math, and beginning writing. Many of the women have experienced some major life crisis, such as divorce, widowhood, economic hardships, or the departure of grown children while many must also deal with severe deficits in their education and training.

The *group for single mothers* meets weekly in two-hour sessions for six to ten weeks. Its five components include support (to decrease isolation through sharing with others in a similar situation), problem-solving (through the selection of one problem and the implementation and monitoring of change strategies for its resolution), education (e.g., parenting skills, stress management), consciousness raising (discussion of the political and social realities for women as single parents) and group leadership training (to establish and maintain ongoing support groups).

*Assertion training classes for women* are attended by those who recognize assertion deficits in themselves and wish to develop new skills. Each of the six weekly sessions is three hours in length and focuses on a particular assertive skill. Though the emphasis is on education and skill development, the connection between women's lack of assertion and their socialization is made amply clear. Parallel with the modeling, rehearsal, and real-life trials of new assertive behaviors, an important component is the explicit permission given for the appropriateness of assertive behavior in women.

Common to all four groups are the considerable age range (18 to 65) and representation across all socio-economic and occupational categories. Some ethnic-minority women participate in each of the groups. Membership ranges from six to twenty-five women; all women are self-selected.

With this brief account of the groups as background, several features they have in common will now be discussed. The literature on other peer-support groups indicate their utility in a wide variety of situations (Powell, 1975; Abramson, 1975; Mantell, 1976) and the supportive, expressive and practical help functions they serve (Schwartz, 1976) are evident in the groups under discussion. However, the particular features emphasized here are those derived from a purposeful feminist stance.

## The End to Women's Particular Isolation

All planned groups deal with isolation to some extent, since their central characteristic is the inclusion of individuals in a group experience. What appears unique to the feminist group is the counteracting of the special isolation which has kept women from valuing each other and understanding their common experiences.

First, the women in some of these groups suffer from special degrees of isolation. For example, the male batterer characteristically holds the woman in a particularly controlled and isolated condition, banning social contacts with friends and relatives, and severely restricting and monitoring ordinary activities outside the home (e.g., shopping, visiting). These women often have no experience with other abused women, have lost almost all contact with other individuals, and consider themselves alone and unique in their situation. Similarly, though for different reasons, many single parents, as they join the group, do not know other single parents. They have neither the time nor resources to seek out others apart from work, and they enter the group feeling that no one else has their problems. Married women who reenter the educational setting report isolation as well.

Though the degree of isolation for other women may be less intense, common to most women is the lack of connection and explicit discussion with other women about the commonalities of their experience in a sexist society. Common to most women also is that they receive and incorporate all their lives societal messages which devalue women in each others' eyes. In the four groups described here, women not only learn (often for the first time) that other women share their circumstances, but they learn to respect and value other women for their intelligence, support, skills, and leadership.

Women enter each of these groups believing not only that they are singularly alone, but that in our society, men hold the power, are to be looked to for problem solving and approval, and that women assume roles of lesser importance or are competitors for men. As examples, women in single-parent groups report that they have few close women friends with whom they can share their concerns, and in fact, express a distrust of women and a sense that they have always preferred to be with and talk to men (Burden, 1980). In the group, they not only meet other women facing the same problems who also need to develop resources within themselves, but for the first time, they come to know and trust other women. The reentering woman in the educational setting can often articulate what her husband or boyfriend wants, but must struggle to discover her own academic and work aspirations. As she works through this process with other women, both her needs and those of other women assume a new importance. Similarly, women in assertion training classes find it initially difficult to identify the areas in which they want to be more assertive because they have been placed in a second-class position vis-a-vis men all their lives and have not permitted their own wishes and plans to surface. Recognizing that the entire arena of women's lives has been devalued creates a new appreciation among the women for their respective needs and capabilities.

In the abused women group, women aware of the abuse in their own lives and of the importance of stopping abuse against all women seem to provide the empathy that bridges the characteristically extreme isolation of battered women. Empathy between such women can foster the interdependency that reduces feelings of dependence on the abusive man. Often asking a group member for her telephone number and information or advice is a first effort to seek help from another woman. The discovery that women can depend on each other for emotional sustenance, as well as expertise in various areas comes as an exciting new learning for many women. Women who have themselves been abused have a special ability to foster such interdependence among women (Nicarthy, 1982).

In all of these groups, participants learn to help each other feel less alone. They realize that their previous isolation from and distrust of other women is largely a social mandate that has kept them from seeing women's competencies as equal to those of men. The end of their isolation has double value as participants are purposefully made aware of the benefits from women's interdependence and helped to take pride in women's accomplishments.

## An Emphasis on Social and Political Factors

Each of the groups introduces in a planned way a societal and political perspective so that women can see that their individual situations are directly related to a variety of larger, social factors. These factors include: (1) the stereotyped socialization of all women, which leads to self-doubts about their competencies and judgment; (2) society's devaluation of women's work both inside and outside the home and social policies which do not provide supports for that work; (3) sexual exploitation and condoned violence throughout our public life resulting in physical abuse and sexual assault.

The curriculum in the women's reentry program is designed to include information on the role and status of women in American society. Socialization of women is part of the college program's module on assertiveness training (as is also true of the separate assertion training classes reported here). The economic factors related to women's lives is introduced in career explorations.

The heterogeneity of each abused women's group dramatizes for every participant the pervasiveness of the problem and its political nature. The individual aspect of abuse is often all the women have previously known. The leaders, as well as some of the group members, specifically place the problem in a political context. Members provide examples of the impact of legal, medical and social policies on their own lives. For instance, official police policy has traditionally been to defuse the "family fight" rather than to arrest the batterer for the crime of assault. Women in the group learn from the leader and each other that tolerance of the abuse of women is a result of official decisions by people in positions of institutional power. In some instances, group members take political action which may begin with individual women acting as each others' advocates in confronting representatives of social institutions, writing letters of protest or by serving as witnesses at hearings for shelter funding.

Awareness of social policy issues is especially useful for single mothers so they can redefine their difficulties in coping as resulting from the low economic status of women in this country and, in particular, from the lack of supportive programs for single parent families rather than from individual personal deficiencies. They learn that occupational segregation relegates 80% of all employed women to low-paid clerical, service, and domestic positions in which they earn less than 60% of men's salaries (Barrett, 1979; Brown, 1976; Kreps & Clark, 1975; Smith, 1979). It takes two wage earners for most husband/wife families to maintain a middle-class lifestyle; single parent women are forced to live on one low income (Burden, 1980; Ross & Sawhill, 1975; Smith, 1979). They see that very few programs exist here that are available in other countries, such as national health care, subsidized child care, and family allowances.

Though each of the groups acknowledges and deals with individual circumstances, facilitators recognize the therapeutic value to the individual woman of understanding that the problem is, to a large extent, the result of cultural mandates or policy decisions.

## *Appropriate Expectations for Individual Responsibility*

There is a two-fold connection between this political stance by the facilitator and the women's individual changes within the group. First, women are enabled to recognize the political aspects of their individual problem and thereby make more rational decisions about what can be individually controlled and what requires political action. Second, based on this understanding, the group process itself fosters realistic changes.

Recognition of the political aspects of personal problems is an important first step in group work with abused women. Their assumption that they are alone in their victimization has contributed to their conviction that they must be at fault. Many women still imagine that only certain types of women—bad, crazy, or inadequate women—are battered or psychologically abused. It is often a dramatic experience for them the first time they attend a group with other abused women to see others who did not fit these stereotypes, and to hear violence discussed as a pervasive social problem.

When reentering college women are first exposed to the general societal picture, the initial reaction is frequently anger. Then they seem determined to change their individual world. They are helped in this effort by a sense of relief that their predicament is not an individual problem alone, but one shared by many women. This larger societal view can change the notion of individual failure, as illustrated by the woman who realizes her avoidance of math, for example, is not due to her incompetence, but to sex-role related assumptions. This realization often frees her to begin her education in math. Realizing that their narrow career choices (e.g., teaching, secretarial, nursing) are culturally induced and may have little to do with individual interests, skills, and abilities, allows women to begin exploring nontraditional occupations and a wider range of careers.

Trainees in assertiveness classes are relieved to know that their more passive stance is not a reflection of individual inadequacy, but of society's expectations for women's behavior. They also begin to understand that they act out those prescribed roles because they have learned and been strongly reinforced for those behaviors. If stereotyped behavior is learned, however, alternate behaviors can also be learned.

Single parents entering groups frequently feel overwhelmed by their responsibilities, but also feel that they should somehow be able to cope with all the demands of childrearing, job, and homemaking. Their sense of the world is that everyone else is managing very well and that they, therefore, must be deficient because life is so difficult for them. They blame themselves for not being able to earn an adequate income, find reasonably priced quality daycare, manage the multiple demands of running a household and maintaining a job, and still have to meet their own social and intimacy needs. Once they recognize that many of their problems are caused by external, often unfair, economic and political factors beyond their immediate control, they begin developing workable strategies to have an impact on their environment to as great an extent as possible. The anger at what they perceive to be an unjust system toward women and children helps them to realize why their situation is so difficult, and to understand that the issue is not individual deficiency. Mobilizing anger frees the women to prioritize their many problems and choose one to work on within the group.

Based on this separation of individual responsibility from the political context, the group process enables women to alter their attitudes and change their situations. A series of typical interactions within the abused women's groups illustrates the impact of the group on the individual woman. Many abused women have been brainwashed into believing that they must obey their husband or boyfriend, that they somehow deserve to be abused, or that they cannot or should not leave the man, yet will become outraged when other women in the group say that they themselves have no right to safety from abuse. When an individual woman hears other women who have experienced similar abuse express helplessness about preventing abuse, she may protest, ''But you're a worthwhile person, you can't let him do that to you!'' When the response to her is then, ''What about you? Why are *you* letting your man do it to you?'', she begins to see that she herself can claim rights she believes others should exercise.

A part of feeling alone and to blame, as an abused woman, is believing that the man is unique in his demeaning treatment. In the group, women are amazed that the men sound so much alike. A ripple of laughter travels around the circle when women hear that other men also ''call every hour from work to check on me,'' or ''check the odometer to see that I haven't been anywhere but the grocery store.'' The implication is that the man, not the woman, is the one who is ''acting crazy.''

Women in relationships with abusive men are sometimes ashamed and embarrassed to express feelings which might be interpreted as weakness. Therapist, relatives, and friends are often impatient with these feelings, in the light of the potential danger. Other women in the group, however, who have been battered and who have virtually all experienced similar feelings, can easily empathize with those feelings, while still encouraging each woman to take the risk of leaving.

Sometimes women cry when they hear others' stories and the tears of empathy convey understanding and caring in a way that very few professionals can provide. Since these women often feel that the only person who cares about them is the very man who abuses them, recognizing that other women care breaks a link in the chain of harmful dependency on one man. At the same time, the links of interdependency among women are strengthened.

In the ongoing drop-in group, women at all stages of abuse and getting-free-of-abuse are exposed to each other. A woman who has just left a dangerous man hears another who has stayed away for weeks or months talk about how the rewards far outweigh the emotional and practical problems. Women who have been in abusive situations for a long time talk about how much worse the abuse has become over the years and about how much harder it is to leave after many years of abuse. Younger women hear them and gain a sense of the probability that their relationship will become more, rather than less, dangerous. Those who have left, but are shaky about staying away, are reminded by other women's stories of what dangers they have escaped. A woman who feels she is "getting nowhere" is reminded by others how much more desperate she was a few weeks before, and how much she has accomplished. Each time one woman encourages another she is reinforcing her own determination to remain free of abuse.

In the assertion training classes, women generally become good coaches for one another, providing useful feedback, as new roles are rehearsed, and realistic reinforcement for successful trials between sessions. Most interesting, however, is the interweaving of their respective abilities. Many women, for example, are more effective in assertiveness in the private sphere and less so in the public ("I can be clear and straightforward with my husband, there's no way I can tell my supervisor I feel exploited."). In most cases, there are counterparts within the same group who have the opposite abilities ("My co-workers and my boss at work are no problem, but telling my husband and my teenagers they need to help more around the house is more than I can imagine doing.''). These differences lead women to be more tolerant of each other as they are learning new skills, and the more successful women in a particular sphere can assist their co-members in that sphere.

## The Absence of Men as Constructive Group Strategy

The primary purpose of all-female memberships in groups is that women need the opportunity to create different and less stereotyped roles for themselves vis-a-vis both women and men, and that attitudes and feelings about themselves as women can find the best arena for expression in all-female environments (Carlock & Martin, 1977). A feminist-oriented atmosphere allows women to develop the meaningful relationships with other women that society ordinarily denies. Examples of the importance of all-female membership will illustrate the point.

Single-parent women who enter their groups frequently express extreme hostility toward men. They are often in the initial post-separation stages or if they have been separated for a long time, are engaged in continual conflict over child support and visitation rights with the children's father. Many women state that they would not have joined the group if there had been men involved. They utilize the first few sessions to ventilate a great deal of anger towards men.

Single parents like most white women in our culture, were socialized to expect to be married and cared for by a man all of their lives. Black women in the groups express a somewhat different socialization experience (i.e., they expect to work outside the home), but they too express great anger towards men (Burden, 1980). Many women are outraged that their expectations have not been fulfilled. They often feel that they fulfilled their side of the bargain and that they were betrayed. For heterosexual women, their sense of self-esteem and image of life in general are strongly dependent on the external factor of the man in their life. Much of the process of the group involves working through with single parents the need to regain an internal locus of control and to take responsibility for their own lives. Also involved is the distinction between interpersonal anger directed at a specific man and political anger at the unfairness of the status of women in our society compared with men. Toward the end of the sessions, women frequently find that their anger towards men and their ex-spouse dissipates somewhat. They may remain angry at the political situation of women while at the same time be able to begin developing friendship and intimacy relationships with both men and women and by the end of the sessions, group members often express the feeling that now they would be ready for a group of both men and women.

In both the college setting and the assertion training classes, facilitators have found that in mixed groups, women defer to men, allow them to take the lead in all discussions, and find it difficult to discover their own values and express their own needs (Baird, 1976). In the abused women's groups, there are special reasons for the inadvisability for the inclusion of men. Not only are men the perpetrators of the abuse women suffer, but as in the single-parent group, their presence would dampen the needed expression of anger. Battered women also experience tremendous feelings of humiliation about admitting the abuse they have suffered. Only in a group of similarly victimized peers are they safe in the knowledge that speaking the unspeakable will reduce their sense of shame, rather than add to it.

## Developing Skills for Ongoing Groups

From the outset in each of the feminist groups, skills are developed that help the individual to gain greater control over her own life and to use the resources of the women's group for support and practical aid. The advantages of the continuing group are first, the provision of a needed psychological and practical support system, and second, the development of a process which enables many women to discover untapped leadership skills.

For many single-parent women, the group is their first such group experience. They initially admit feeling intimidated by the group and fearful of speaking in front of so many people. An important benefit of the group is the leadership training provided. After the first two sessions, members increasingly assume responsibility for the direction of the group. They identify issues they want to discuss from week to week, and they report on their problem-solving projects. From the beginning, the option of continuing the group on their own as a friendship/support group is discussed. Ongoing groups are usually formed by members who live geographically close to each other. Using the original group leader as an occasional consultant, groups may continue to meet once or twice a month on their own for several years.

As an outcome of the women's class in the reentering women's program, women study together and assist each other in a number of other practical situations as they continue their education. Encouraged to develop leadership skills some women also choose to use those skills in student government, advisory boards, and other positions of leadership.

The assertion training leader purposefully and explicitly describes all aspects of the skills program at each point along the way so that the participants are aware that they can easily assemble for themselves the components of a group program for continued learning. From the beginning the leader promotes the idea of a continuing group to reinforce skills developed in the initial training as well as to provide new learning. Usually at the final session, a continuing group is formed, sometimes with a planned occasional consultation by the facilitator, but more often with a proposed, completely self-directed group.

Built into the group process in work with abused women are the elements of a continuing support network outside the group. A time is set aside during each of the sessions for the exchange of telephone numbers in that each woman has several others to call when she is lonely, fearful or tempted to return to the man who battered her. A myriad of practical problems face any woman who is separating from any man—housing, money, child care, and employment problems. These problems are compounded by the necessity for legal advice, for secrecy in living quarters, and for recovery from emotional and physical trauma. The facilitator can provide resource information, but half a dozen or more women who have "been there" can be far more informative and creative.

## CONCLUSION

The themes which characterize these groups are by their very nature the distinctive qualities of all-women feminist groups. Women will develop a solidarity among themselves when they do not have to consider another set of issues which occur by virtue of the presence of men. That particular solidarity—created around women's potential to overcome stereotypes—will develop more effectively when a feminist interpretation has been offered by the facilitators. Women will be more likely to end their true isolation from each other, understand the political import of their status, and develop particular individual and group skills when facilitators attend specifically to these issues.

These themes are not exhaustive of the group experience. The question remains whether feminist-oriented groups are more effective for the women participants than other groups might be. There is some evidence of long-term gains for some of these efforts (Richey, 1981) but we are not aware of studies which specifically compare a feminist orientation with other frameworks for the group process.

We believe, however, that there is enough experience in feminist groups over many years and across groups with different purposes at least to raise some questions for those offering other groups to women. Is sufficient attention paid to the effects on women of a mixed-sex group? Can a group experience for women (or for that matter any service) be effective which does not actively attempt to surmount harmful stereotypes or does not purposefully increase the control women can assume over their own lives? Experience to date in these feminist groups is sufficient to invite facilitators of mixed-sex or non-feminist women's groups to consider whether their approaches are meeting women's needs sufficiently.

## REFERENCES

Abramson, M. Group treatment of burn-injured patients. *Social Casework,* 1975, *56,* 235-241.

Baird, J. Sex differences in group communication: A review of relevant research. *Quarterly Journal of Speech,* 1976, *62,* 179-192.

Barrett, N. Women in the job market: Occupations, earnings, and career opportunities. In R. E. Smith (ed.) *The Subtle Revolution: Women at Work.* Washington, D.C.: The Urban Institute, 1979.

Brown, G. How type of employment affects earnings differences by sex. *Monthly Labor Review,* 1976, *99,* 25-30.

Burden, D. Women as single parents: Alternative services for a neglected population. In N. Gottlieb (ed.) *Alternative Social Services for Women,* New York: Columbia University Press, 1980.

Carlock, C. and Martin, P. Sex composition and the intensive group experience, *Social Work,* 1977, *22,* 27-33.

Kreps, J. and Clark, R. *Sex, age and work: The changing composition of the labor force.* Baltimore: Johns Hopkins University Press, 1975.

Mantell, J., Alexander, E., and Klerman, M. Social work and self-help groups. *Health and Social Work,* 1976, *1,* 86-100.

Nicarthy, G. *Getting Free,* Seattle: Seal Press, 1982.

Powell, T. The use of self-help groups as supportive reference communities. *American Journal of Orthopsychiatry,* 1975, *45,* 756-764.

Richey, C. Assertiveness training for women. In S. Schinke (ed.) *Behavioral Methods in Social Welfare.* New York: Aldine, 1981.

Ross, H. and Sawhill, I. *Time of transition: The growth of families headed by women.* Washington, D.C.: The Urban Institute.

Schwartz, M. Situation/transition groups: A conceptualization and review. *American Journal of Orthopsychiatry,* 1976, *45,* 744-755.

Smith, R. (ed.) *The subtle revolution: Women at work.* Washington, D.C.: The Urban Institute, 1979.

# Call for Papers

Contributions are invited for a special issue of *Social Work with Groups*. The edition is to appear in the Fall of 1985 and will be devoted entirely to group work with children and adolescents. Special editors will be James Garland and Ralph Kolodny of Boston University. Consideration will be given to both theoretical and descriptive articles. This includes presentations which discuss the opportunities and limitations in special approaches, as well as ethnic, class and gender variations as they affect work with groups of this age. Papers which deal with the impact of setting on practice with children and youth are likewise eagerly sought. Original papers on any and all aspects of the topic are welcome.

All manuscripts should conform to the requirements of manuscripts for *Social Work with Groups*. They can be submitted to the special editors of this issue at Boston University School of Social Work, 264 Bay State Rd., Boston, Mass. 02215.

# Managing Conflict
# in All-Women Groups

## Beverly Hartung Hagen

**ABSTRACT.** Due to the influence of the women's movement with its early emphasis on consciousness-raising groups, all-women groups have become increasingly utilized for a broad spectrum of purposes including counselling, drug dependence treatment, assertiveness training, and mutual support. As a result, an increasing amount of literature on all-women groups is being generated, but very little focuses on the issue of conflict as either a developmental stage or a specific entity in all-women groups.

This paper will explore the following issues having to do with all-women groups and conflict: (1) early socialization of women regarding conflict, (2) reasons why conflict is an especially difficult subject for most women, (3) information to share with women about conflict and suggestions for attitudinal and educational exercises, (4) strategies for arbitration if conflict becomes problematic.

The small group as a vehicle for support and individual change has been used effectively by social workers and other helping profession practitioners for many years. We have learned that all groups must find ways to use differences among members productively, develop decision making procedures and a common view of the group's task, decide on working roles and procedures, and maintain a mutually satisfying balance between meeting member needs and addressing a group's goals. All of these tasks require a group to grapple with potential conflict and control issues among members.

All-women groups were initially formed for purposes of consciousness raising (CR), support, and social change during the early stages of the current women's movement. Increasingly, practitioners are recognizing the value of the all-women groups for many

Beverly Hartung Hagen is Assistant Professor, School of Social Work, University of Nebraska at Omaha, Omaha, NE 68182-0293.

types of problems, practice situations, and purposes. As more experience is gained and research conducted in all-women groups,
however, it is becoming apparent that all-women groups differ in
many ways from groups with male members. Issues related to
handling conflict and control within the group appear to be particularly problematic. How an all-women group approaches these
issues is affected by the purpose of the group, the ideology members
bring to it, the nature of women's socialization and experience, and
perhaps even by differences in the progression of developmental
stages within the group.

Special attention to dealing with conflict and control issues will be
important in most or all types of all-women groups (especially those
with a feminist orientation), but is likely to be especially important
in CR groups. Most women join CR groups to find a supportive atmosphere in which they can discuss their experiences being female
in a sexist society. The CR group's goals of openness and support
and its traditional deemphasis of formal leadership can effectively
facilitate this effort if the group can work through the issues of conflict and control that researchers and theorists have observed to be a
part of the group process.

The purpose of this paper is to discuss the following areas: (1)
reasons why conflict and control are likely to be especially difficult
areas in all-women groups; (2) strategies group leaders, consultants, and members might use to help group members accept and
value their differences; (3) development of norms and skills for
managing conflict and power issues in productive ways.

## ALL-WOMEN GROUPS AND CONFLICT

### The Development and Dynamics
### of All-Women Groups

Most theories and research on group development and functioning suggest that some degree of interpersonal conflict is likely, in
fact necessary, if the group is to perform well, use its members'
resources effectively, and achieve a satisfactory level of intimacy
among members. Although they are not in total agreement about the
number and names of group stages, group theorists and researchers
contend that developmental stages are experienced by all types of
groups regardless of their structure and functions (e.g., Yalom,
1976; Thelen & Dickerman, 1974; Garland, Jones, & Kolodny,

1973; Mackey, 1980). At least one of these stages is characterized by high degrees of conflict among members and concerns about power and control. Negotiating this stage effectively and developing norms and procedures for addressing these issues are necessary if the group is to move into deeper levels of intimacy and/or more effective working procedures.

Most of the research on group development and member behaviors, however, has occurred in groups that include men. Much less is known about all-women groups and how they develop and function. Until definitive studies of all-women groups are conducted to ascertain the role, if any, developmental stages play in these groups, the question remains as to whether same-sex groups also pass through developmental stages and if so, whether or not these stages are the same as in mixed groups.

Some observers of all-women groups do mention a stage which is defined, in part, by focus on issues of conflict and control. After observing a women's group over a period of time, Eastman (1973) described a stage in which conflict occurred when a split developed between women who wanted to use the group to form close relationships and those who wanted to maintain a distance. At that point, the temporary leaders encouraged ventilation. Eastman later observed "four stages of sharing, opening up, analyzing, and abstracting occurred kaleidoscopically and unevenly with different women able to hook in and become engaged at various points" (p. 170). Other authors have also described the progression of all-women groups toward cohesion. In some, conflicts that emerged were successfully negotiated (e.g., Sanford, 1979) and in others, they were not (e.g., Patlee, 1977).

These descriptions also suggest that all-women groups may move through developmental stages somewhat differently than do group with men members. In general, all-women groups appear to begin working on intimacy and interpersonal issues earlier than groups that include men, tending also to do this more intensely and directly than in mixed groups. In fact, conflict may not surface until members begin to feel some degree of knowledge about each other and a fairly high degree of trust and safety. This sequence, compared to mixed group development, may mean that in all-women groups, work in norms about intimacy and personal relationships becomes entangled with work on developing leadership procedures and group structures appropriate and comfortable for the members of the group. Thus, there may be more confusion among these issues, and group members may experience differences related to procedures and task-orientation as indications of an unwillingness to disclose or be close, or even as personal rejection.

One of the consequences of this confusion about differences may be an avoidance of conflict in all-women groups. Aries (1977) reports that women in all-women groups tended not to deal with competition and aggression issues, discussing subjects such as loving others, home, and family instead. Carlock and Martin (1977) found that women competed with each other very little in all-women groups, choosing instead to intellectualize on the subject of competition in a way they believed worked through the competition issue. This was in contrast with the competitive feelings they reported towards each other for the attention of men in mixed groups.

All of this is complicated by an ideology common in many feminist groups (for CR and other purposes) explicitly rejecting confrontation, conflict, and competition as undesirable aspects of male-defined interpersonal relationships and hierarchies. Several authors have addressed some of the difficulties that can arise from this perspective carried to an extreme (e.g., Joreen, 1973; Crow, Riddle, & Sparks, 1978). The special emphasis given to process and interpersonal support may mean that different orientations to group outcomes or products are experienced as personal conflicts, and the deemphasis of traditional forms of leadership may lead to covert power struggles and an increasing inability for anyone to provide constructive leadership.

On the other hand, in many all-women groups, the work that has occurred to develop supportive norms, cooperation, and a more egalitarian status structure has led to flexible democratic models of leadership as well as structures that allow members to contribute leadership and other resources as they feel able. In addition, Tuddenham, MacBride, and Zahn (1958) found that women tend to conform more in mixed groups than in same sex groups, implying that women were more able to stand up for themselves with other women. This increased assertiveness and individuality also can lead to more possibilities for disagreement, conflict, or confrontation with each other.

## Women's Socialization and Interpersonal Orientation

A search of the literature having to do with conflict and confrontation reveals that there is very little information about how women work through conflicts with one another. Some writers do discuss women and anger in general. Wykoff (1977) states, "We are told not to show our anger, sadness, pain, or hatred, not aware in the process of suppressing these emotions we loose our capacity to feel love, joy and ecstacy. When we cut off our so called negative feelings, we also limit our positive ones" (p. 35).

Many of us also can recall as children having been told that anger wasn't "lady-like" or that "little girls shouldn't get mad." Along with such traditional admonitions, many little girls have not been taught how to deal with angry feelings on a personal or social level or how to effectively identify anger or conflict describing such feelings as hurt or disappointment. As a result, many women also tend to cry rather than shout, or experience pain rather than express anger.

In a somewhat different but related vein, Bardwick (1977) postulates that women do not like to be seen as powerful as they believe power requires more responsibility and more negative consequences from its possessor. On the other hand, Bardwick sees powerlessness as producing anxiety and therefore anger-provoking. With such a combination, the possibility of a group of women working together over a long period of time in a group setting without experiencing occasional conflict with each other is quite unlikely.

Even if it is true that both men and women see conflict as something to be avoided, women still are at a decided disadvantage socially and emotionally when called upon to manage conflict with each other. First, conflict is often seen in our society as a distancing behavior, one which easily would result in rejection and/or abandonment. Since women have been socialized to value support and depend on others to fulfill many emotional needs, the perceived consequence of rejection or abandonment could be a powerful deterrent to confronting conflict. Secondly, inexperience in the whole area of power and conflict could lead an all-women group to remain in beginning stages of group development until the group terminates or could also result in a mixed group continuing to wrestle with issues prominent in earlier stages of group development. This is important because much of the research on mixed groups indicates that it is through such openness about conflict that groups acquire the capacity to move toward increased cohesiveness and productivity.

Finally, early parental admonitions about anger, fear of rejection, and lack of experience with conflict may cause women to misjudge the nature of conflict in the conflict and power stage of groups. If women perceive conflict in this stage as a personal assault rather than an inevitable progression or if they believe conflict is a sign of a troubled group rather than a healthy one, they may also be tempted to remain in the polite, intellectualized, but superficial stage of the beginning group, thereby preventing the group from attaining the cohesion necessary to attain their individual and/or group goals.

## STRATEGIES FOR FACILITATING CONFLICT MANAGEMENT IN ALL-WOMEN GROUPS

### Before the Conflict Arises

Many of these strategies will also be helpful even after a group has encountered a conflict situation, but in general, it is usually less painful and more efficient to anticipate that difficulties with power and conflict may arise and help a group develop norms, skills, and procedures that will enable it to use its conflict constructively. How this can be accomplished depends on a number of factors, among them a person's role in the group. If you are the group's designated leader, you can plan activities early that will facilitate later constructive use of conflict. If you are a member, and the group is leaderless, you could share with the group the information contained in this paper, and suggest including some of these "prevention" activities early in its life together. A group can also contract with a consultant knowledgeable in dealing with problems in the conflict area.

*Educational sessions.* Since many women have been taught during childhood that they are not to be powerful (and this is often reinforced by society during adulthood), one of the first issues that will probably be considered will be that of the inevitability of power and influence in all human interaction. Once group members realize that all human beings have power and influence in relation to each other and that the exercise of such power is an integral part of cooperation, the group should be more ready to deal with individual power and conflict issues.

Women also need to realize that power is an infinite commodity which is personal. We do not take each other's power, nor does the powerfulness of one woman diminish the power of another. As Bardwick hypothesized: "They (women) seem to see power as being limited. Either one has it or not; and if one person has it, then another cannot" (1977, p. 328). Exploration of the differences between power and manipulation (power, a natural attribute we each possess; manipulation, a type of shrewd control of others in an unfair or dishonest way) should also help group members look at power as a component of cooperation and help them approach and deal with whatever conflicts and disagreements that might arise.

Johnson and Johnson relate group effectiveness to conflict management, stating that many groups are less effective because they do not examine their procedures and their relevance to the needs and goals of both the members of the group and also the world itself (pp. 203-231). They continue by stating that conflicts have the potential for encouraging both personal and group change and can revitalize existing group practices. If, therefore, an all-women group is able to see conflicts in such a positive light, such an attitude in and of itself may be sufficient to help a group work through whatever they need to enable to reach the cohesion at work stages.

*Group exercises.* One way women might use to practice dealing with differences could be group games or structured exercises which focus on an awareness of conflict and how each woman tries to influence others. One such exercise instructs the participants to divide into groups of three with each woman identifying herself as A, B, or C. A is then told to try to convince B to do something with her or for her. B is to carefully consider A's proposal and then decide what to do. C is to observe and give feedback on techniques A used to influence others. Members must then switch roles until each woman has experienced each role. Discussion in this exercise will probably center around how each woman uses influence, the type of influence she chooses, what was found to be the most convincing technique of influencing others, and how she felt about trying to influence others.

A number of other exercises are also possible and could be useful depending on the group. Values clarification tasks with interpersonal relationships, conflict and power issues, leadership definitions and values, incorporated into them can be very helpful (e.g., Wedenoja & Reed, 1982). Non-verbal exercises in which people try to practice expressing anger, submission, dominance, etc. can also be very thought provoking.

*Practice in interpersonal communication and feedback techniques.* A range of techniques are available for teaching and practicing interpersonal and communication skills (cf., Pfeiffer & Jones, annual). Introducing guidelines for, and practice in, giving effective feedback is a particularly useful tool (Wedenoja & Reed, 1982; Auvine, Densmore, Extrom, Poole, & Shanklin, 1978; Lyons, 1976; Manis, 1977; Johnson & Johnson, 1977). In brief, these guidelines suggest the following: (1) feedback is specific rather than general, (2) feedback describes rather than judges, (3) feedback is directed toward behavior that the receiver can do something about, (4) feedback is tentative rather than absolute, (5) feedback informs rather than commands or accuses, (6) feedback is asked for rather than imposed, (7) feedback clarifies expectations and requests, (8) feedback is direct, (9) feedback is checked to be sure that the listener hears and understands (Wedenoja & Reed, pp. 100-101). The authors continue by suggesting that these guidelines can be learned and applied through leader modeling, structured exercises, role plays, etc. Other types of interpersonal skills education such as assertiveness training could also be very productively taught and applied in all-women groups.

## After the Conflict Arises

All of the above can also be useful after the fact, but may take longer and be more stressful for group members. Some conflicts may also be unresolvable—after all, even good people do not always agree or think exactly alike. In this case, if the group can not work the conflict through, a group consultant or arbitrator may be able to help the group address the conflict in such a way that the group remains viable and intact. Some possible roles in the intervention of a third party in conflict are described by Morton Deutsch (1973) who suggests the following possible roles of an arbitrator in such a situation.

(1) Identification and confrontation of the issues. Sometimes the mere presence of the third party may lessen anxiety, change motivation, and alter the power structure. (2) Creation of an atmosphere which is conducive to conflict resolution. This can be done by selecting a mutually satisfactory meeting place, setting the pace of discussion by regulating the tension, encouraging creative and productive actions, etc. (3) Removal of communication blocks or distortions to facilitate mutual understanding. (4) Establishment of rules of productive interaction such as mutual respect and open communication. In this situation, the arbitrator helps parties to fight fair and set fair rules, avoid moralism, generalizing, or issuing ultimatums or threats. Rules need to be as unbiased as possible. (5) Determination of solutions which are both possible and productive. The arbitrator needs to help the group members discover their aspirations and expectations of each party, also helping the members

deal with those which are unrealistic or impossible. (6) Encourage a workable agreement acceptable to the parties in conflict. This also involves helping each party to the conflict save face and feel good about the final agreement. (7) Insure that both the negotiations and the final agreement seem prestigeful and attractive to the interested audience and the group itself. This makes it more likely that both the parties of the conflict and the group will be satisfied with the outcome of the conflict.

## CONCLUDING REMARKS

All-women groups can serve very important functions for their members and have also accomplished significant social changes over the past ten years. Group goals and structures vary from political activities, to mostly social activities, to intense emotional interaction. The difficulties that these groups have with conflict and power can keep them from realizing their full potential for helping women deal with mutual problems of living in a male-dominated world. We have stated that conflict is probably an integral part of group process for all-women groups, although its timing and form may differ from what is observed in all-men or mixed groups. Understanding and anticipating this fact, and the likely benefits to be had if it can be used constructively, should help potential members and leaders of such groups to minimize the negative effects of conflict and move towards developing even more flexible and resourceful group structures and processes.

The issue of leadership must be considered carefully when thinking about how best to facilitate conflict management in any given situation. A "leaderless" form of group such as the traditional CR group may need to move towards a more designated leader situation as the group moves toward more action oriented behavior. "Small groups began with the basic premise of equality. When the focus of groups shifted from CR to action, these concepts were called into question" (Jenkins & Kramer, 1978, p. 74). On the other hand, a strong leader or co-leader in the initial stages of a group can help it develop an atmosphere, skills, norms, and clear goals and procedures so that the group is able to move towards a situation of much more shared leadership over time. In either case, denying or pretending that conflict doesn't exist, or avoiding it, or labeling it, or the people experiencing it as bad, can only lead a group into more and more difficulty.

# REFERENCES

Aries, E. Interaction patterns and themes of male, female and mixed groups. *Small Group Behavior,* 1976, *7,* 7-18.

Auvine, B., Densmore, B., Extrom, M., Poole, S., & Shanklin, M. *A Manual for Group Facilitators.* Available from The Center for Conflict Resolution, 731 State Street, Madison, Wis. 53703, 1978.

Bardwick, J. M. Some notes about power relationships between women. In A. Sargent (Ed.), *Beyond Sex Roles.* St. Paul, Minn., West Publishing House, 1977.

Carlock, C. J. & Martin, P. Y. Sex composition and the intensive group experience. *Social Work,* 1977, *22,* 27-32.

Crow, G. The process/product split. *Quest,* 1978, *4,* 15-23.

Deutsch, M. *The Resolution of Conflict, Constructive and Destructive Processes.* New Haven & London: Yale University Press, 1973.

Eastman, P. C. Consciousness-raising as a resocialization process for women. *Smith College Studies in Social Work,* 1973, *43,* 153-183.

Garland, J., Jones, H., & Kolodny, R. A model for stages of development in social work groups. In S. Berstein (Ed.), *Explorations in Group Work.* Kennebunkport, Maine: Milford House, 1973.

Jenkins, L. & Kramer, C. Small group process: Learning from women. *Women's Studies International Quarterly,* 1978, *1,* 67-84.

Johnson, D. W. & Johnson, F. P. *Joining Together: Group Theory and Group Skills.* New Jersey: Prentice-Hall, Inc., 1983.

Joreen. The tyranny of structurelessness. In Koedt, A., Levine, E., & Rapone, A., (Eds.), *Radical Feminism.* New York: Quadrangle Books, 1973, 285-299.

Lyons, G. *Constructive Criticism: A Handbook.* Available from Issues in Radical Therapy Collective, P.O. Box 23544, Oakland, Calif. 94623, 1976.

Mackey, R. A. Developmental process in growth-oriented groups. *Social Work,* 1980, *25,* 26-29.

Manis, L. *Woman Power: A Manual for Workshops in Personal Effectiveness.* Crawston, R.I.: Carroll Press, 1977.

Pottee, C. Organizers' dialogue. *Quest,* 1977, *4,* 26-39.

Pfeiffer, W. J. & Jones, J. E. *Annual Handbook for Group Facilitators.* Available from University Associate, 7596 Eades Avenue, LaJolla, Calif. 92037.

Riddle, D. Integrating process and product. *Quest,* 1978, *4,* 23-32.

Sanford, W. C. Working together growing together. *Heresieo,* 1979, *2,* 83-92.

Sparks, C. Process/product split: A misnomer. *Quest,* 1978, *4,* 32-36.

Thelen, H. & Dickerman, W. Stereotypes and the growth of groups. *Selected Reading Series,* Washington D. C.: National Training Laboratories, National Educational Association, 1974, pp. 73-80.

Tuddenham, R. D., MacBride, & Zahn, V. The influence of the sex composition of the group upon yielding to a distorted norm. *Journal of Psychology,* 1958, *46,* 243-251.

Wedenoja, M., & Reed, B. G. Women's groups as a form of intervention for drug dependent women. In B. G. Reed, G. M. Beschner, & Mondanaro (Eds.), *Treatment Services for Drug Dependent Women* (Vol. 2), Rockville, MD.: National Institute on Drug Abuse, (D.H.H.S. Publication No. A & M 82-1319), 1982.

Wykoff, H. *Solving Women's Problems Through Awareness, Action and Contact.* New York: Grove Press, 1977.

Yalom, I. D. *The Theory and Practice of Group Psychotherapy.* New York: Basic Books, 1975.

# Re-Examining Women's Roles:
# A Feminist Group Approach
# to Decreasing Depression in Women

Monika J. Haussmann
Judith H. Halseth

**ABSTRACT.** Depression in rural women is a problem of epidemic proportions. Within the parameters of a rural mental health center, a feminist group can assist women in examining depressogenic socialization messages. In this 13-week women's group, the focus shifted from a semi-structured socio-educational approach to the participants taking an increasingly active role in bringing in and working on relevant personal concerns. Crucial in the process were re-examining women's role expectations, challenging role-stereotypes, expressing anger, and bonding and networking with each other. The group fostered self-respect, awareness of choices, and assertiveness in previously depressed rural women.

This paper presents the theoretical context, rationale, participants, structure, content, process, and outcome of a thirteen-week group for depressed women in a rural area in Michigan.

## I. Context

Depression is an extremely frequent phenomenon in the United States (Fields, 1980). More women are depressed than are men; estimates as to the exact ratio range from 2:1 to 10:1 (Radloff, Note

At the time of leading this group, both authors were employed at Van Buren County Community Mental Health, Paw Paw, Michigan. Monika J. Haussmann is a psychologist at this agency, and a member of the American Psychological Association. Her mailing address is 5910 C Briarcliff Path, Kalamazoo, MI 49009. Judith H. Halseth, ACSW, is an Assistant Professor of Social Work, and Rural Mental Health Project Director, at the School of Social Work, Western Michigan University, Kalamazoo, Michigan. She is a member of the National Association of Social Workers and the Council on Social Work Education. This is a slightly revised version of a paper printed in the *Proceedings of the Sixth National Institute on Social Work in Rural Areas*, Columbia, SC: Univ. of South Carolina College of Social Work, 1982.

1; Weissman & Klerman, 1977). Theoretical explanations regarding the prevalence of depression in women encompass genetic and endocrinological factors, depressogenic variables in women's socialization process, the learned helplessness model, the cognitive model of depression, effects of marital and occupational roles, and actual social discrimination against women.

The socialization process for most women encourages nurturant, submissive, and conservative aspects of the female role, whereas assertiveness, achievement orientation, and independence are explicitly discouraged (Block, Von der Lippe, & Block, 1973). Daughters, more so than sons, continue affiliations and dependencies well into adulthod (Hoffman, 1975). Women learn to vicariously achieve through their husband's and children's accomplishments rather than through their own (Lipman-Blumen & Leavitt, 1978). They tend to be submissive to a male-dominant-other, and become economically, socially, and psychologically dependent (Arieti, 1979). Due to actual social discrimination, women have difficulties in achieving mastery, direct action, and self-assertion, which may lead to increased vulnerability to loss and to clinical depression (Weissman, 1980). Depressed individuals were found to view themselves as more responsible, in interpersonal rather than impersonal contexts, than nondepressed individuals (Rizley, 1978). High interpersonal responsibility for others' behavior was found to be more typical for women than for men (Alper, 1978). Traditional female roles of wife and mother may contribute to depression (Bernard, 1973; Radloff, 1975).

The combination of these vulnerability variables to depression—lack of direct achievement, high interpersonal responsibility, little actual power and status, psychological submissiveness to a dominant-other plus economic dependency, and traditional sex-role attitudes—may partially account for why so many women are depressed in Western cultures.

## II. Treatment Approaches

Rural low-income women are especially vulnerable to depression due to lack of social and educational opportunities, inadequate resources in childcare, transportation difficulties, isolation, and traditional family role demands regardless of a woman's employment. Traditional approaches in the treatment of depression consist of medication and individual psychotherapy; though potentially helpful on a short-term basis, these approaches do little to prevent women's depression which may be due more to societal inequities than to personal failures (Weissman, Note 2).

Many community health centers are not yet designed to facilitate education and prevention; instead, they are often structured according to the medical model in dealing with individuals, with little consideration for larger societal components in a person's distress. Our concern was how we as mental health practitioners could assist women in decreasing depression within the parameters of a rural community mental health setting.

In a recent survey in Michigan, depression in women was found to be associated with perceiving one's partner as dominant, having a low sense of mastery and power, relying on others for achievement, blaming oneself for others' difficulties, and, if employed, having stereotypical attitudes toward women's roles (Haussmann, Notes 3 & 4). These factors are learned through sex-typed female socialization. They can be re-examined and unlearned.

A variety of approaches can facilitate such unlearning through a re-examination of women's roles: (1) Assertiveness training can counteract patterns of helplessness and submissiveness; women learn to challenge socialization messages and to develop a belief system about their personal rights (Butler, 1976). (2) Cognitive approaches can facilitate a rational examination of one's own assumptions and those of others about women's roles. Thus, women can acquire self-reliance, and learn to distance themselves from cultural prejudices (Beck & Greenberg, 1974). (3) Consciousness raising groups can facilitate the exploration of identity issues, and can help women move from personal individual solutions to group actions (Kravetz, 1980). Women resocialize themselves and each other through role-modeling, opening-up, sharing, analyzing, and abstracting from their personal experiences (Kirsh, 1974). (4) Feminist therapists emphasize societal and personal changes rather than adjustment to the status quo. They view the therapist-client relationship as egalitarian; techniques are employed that enhance a client's sense of personal power, self-nurturance, and ability to express anger. The therapist serves as a role model and uses appropriate self-disclosure (Gilberg, 1980). (5) When dealing with women who have no or very little income, real life problems of economic survival have to be addressed through vocational training programs (Messer & Lehrer, 1976). Re-entry of women into school, training programs or employment is a normal transitional stage; support groups are needed in dealing with problems of low self-confidence, role conflict and resulting guilt, and time management (Brooks, 1976). Manis and Mochizuki (1972) developed a Search For Fulfillment program at the Western Michigan University Counseling Center to help re-entry homemakers remove psychological blocks which prevent them from changing their lives. This program consists of trustbuilding, realistic assessment of one's own abilities and of available opportunities in the community, decision-making skills, and risk-taking. (6) All-women groups are likely to be more effective than individual therapy or mixed-sex groups because women then tend to become less dependent on one person, and they learn to receive and give support and protection from and to other women (Carter, 1977).

The facilitators decided to offer an all-women group, based on feminist principles, and designed to decrease depression. The group consisted of an examination of women's roles, assertiveness training, consciousness raising, and mutual support.

## III. Group Participants

The group for depressed women was sponsored by Van Buren County Community Mental Health, Paw Paw, Michigan, Van Buren County is a rural county in Southwestern Michigan, with agriculture, fruit farming and wineries among the main sources of employment. The population is 66,000, and the largest town has 6,000 inhabitants. Approximately 20% of the county residents receive some form of welfare. About 11% of the residents are black, and there is a significant seasonal and "settled-out" migrant population of Mexican-Americans and whites. There are more female clients than male clients at Van Buren County Community Mental Health, and many of the women clients are depressed.

In order to meet the needs of these depressed women, the facilitators designed a group, "Coping with Depression." The group was planned to last for seven weeks (two hours, one evening a week) and was expanded to 13 weeks at the clients' request. The 14 group participants were all clients at Van Buren County Community Mental Health. The facilitators encouraged other agency staff to refer women who were presently depressed, had some communication skills, and were not overtly psychotic at the time of the referral. Eleven participants had been seen individually by the co-facilitators.

Because no minority women participated, it is not known which parts of this group model would be effective with minority women. The mean age of the participants was 35. All had been married at one time; all had children; and all except one were economically dependent on a husband or on ADC. Most of the women had completed high school, and their job skills and experiences were minimal.

## IV. Group Structure, Content, and Process

The co-facilitators' roles were to be responsive to the needs of individuals and the group, to suggest group activities, to provide resource materials, and to participate fully in the group activities. By listening, being supportive, and offering feedback, the co-facilitators served as role models for open communication.

Before the first group meeting, materials and themes were developed and collected. The facilitators both, for the first time, conducted a group specifically designed to assist women in coping with depression. Therefore, they allowed two hours for emotional preparation immediately prior to each group meeting, in addition to ample preparation time during the week, and debriefing time after each meeting. The two-hour time period prior to the meeting helped the facilitators relax, gain a break from a full day's work as individual therapists, and focus on the past week's group meeting. The plan for each specific session was developed week by week in order to be responsive to the needs and energy flow of the participants.

Basic materials used each session included easel and chart paper, marking pens, 3 x 5 cards, and pencils. The women sat in an open circle of chairs. Each session began with an "opener" of an incomplete sentence such as "During the past week I felt depressed (or happy, or sad) when. . ." In this and all other activities, participation was voluntary. The closure each week was also structured to encourage quieter women to participate. Open ended statements were posted including "Tonight I learned. . .," "I was pleased. . .," and "I was displeased. . ." (Manis, Lockwood, Nutter, Mochizuki, & Pattison, 1977).

Brainstorming was frequently used, followed by posting of the ideas on chart paper and processing the feelings and the learning (Pfeiffer & Jones, 1979). Brief lectures and handouts were given on socialization messages girls and women receive (Jakubowski, 1977), depression (Gilmore, 1973), assertiveness (Manis, 1979), anger

(Bienvenu, 1976; Jones & Banet, 1976), and sexuality. Short home-work assignments were given at many sessions.

A refreshment break each week encouraged mutual contact and support. Information was shared on community resources and women's activities. There was discussion of the value of continuing education and of paid employment outside the home. A book table was used one evening to display the facilitators' favorite books on women's development, assertiveness, and sexuality.

During the first seven weeks the activities were semistructured. The women brainstormed, posted and processed the themes, "What we mean when we say 'I'm depressed' ''; "Why people get depressed"; and "Why *women* get depressed." From individual and personal goals, group goals were developed, with the following themes emerging: (a) understand depression, (b) get support and reassurance from the group that I'm not always wrong, (c) learn to stop feeling apologetic or guilty for asking or expecting partner to share responsibilities.

Anger was a significant issue for many women, and some were able to move from being afraid to feel or express anger toward allowing themselves choices about expressing anger in a variety of ways. Assertiveness, aggressiveness, and nonassertiveness were defined (Lange & Jakubowski, 1976), and the women encouraged each other to move assertively toward getting some of their own needs and rights met without violating the needs and rights of others. They discovered that they had rights which they had allowed others but not themselves; they learned to give themselves permission to nurture themselves, and to speak in more positive terms about themselves.

After the first seven sessions, most participants expressed a strong desire to continue the group. Suggestions for improvement of the group were to allow more time to examine one's own difficulties, to role-play more problem situations as they occur at home, and to spend more time sharing, discussing, and integrating new learning.

Therefore, the facilitators designed the next sessions to work in depth on individual concerns, and kept structure and materials to a minimum. The group as a whole was expected to bring up and deal with highly personal issues. The utmost importance of confidentiality was reaffirmed. Participants dealt with a wide variety of intimate issues, and shared previously kept family and personal secrets. The initial enthusiasm and risk-taking was followed by a session characterized by anxiety and withdrawal. The women examined the crucial question whether they could trust each other. Following this probing period, group members worked on problems with single-mothering, unequal power-distribution in one's marriage, value conflicts regarding women's roles, and the "empty nest" experience. From this work, the sense of trust and safety within the group re-emerged. A commonly shared theme surfaced: the exploration of societal double standards regarding expectations of women and men. The group posted two lists, "A Good Woman Should. . .," and "A Good Man Should. . ." The group was amazed and concerned with the results.

For the "good woman," 37 expectations were listed such as "put him first, let the man win, do as he says, always ask permission, not get sick—stay on feet even when sick, keep husband happy. . ." For the "good man," only 10 expectations were listed, such as "not use all his money for his wants, show his feelings more, communicate with wife, take interest in children." The group discussed how attempting to fulfill the impossible masses of "good-woman-expectations" would make anyone depressed. The women realized the importance of developing realistic self-expectations based on one's own needs and wants, rather than living in an attempt to fulfill others' expectations.

The poster on the wall, a quote by Jean Baker Miller (1976), received renewed understanding and importance:

It is only when the woman can move away
from thinking first of pleasing another
and conforming to his desires and expectations
that she can even begin to know herself. (p. 110)

The women worked on affirming their rights as individuals, explored career and lifestyle choices and options, and built increased assertiveness. They became aware of and confronted their tendencies to decrease their positive sense of self by discounting compliments and acknowledgements. Themes of gaining self-respect emerged: accepting and expressing feelings, owning pride in one's accomplishments, and understanding and choosing how to deal with one's anger.

The participants recognized the sense of freedom that comes from taking charge of one's own life rather than asking one's partner to do so. Throughout the group, women were building an informal network system with each other, and planned ways of continuing these networks. When the group closed after 13 sessions, the women noted an increased sense of personal power and a significant decrease in depression and helplessness. This resulted from a sense of belonging and trust in their value as women, individually as well as a group.

## V. Outcome

Ten weeks after termination of the group, the facilitators mailed a group-evaluation form. Excerpts from the members' written evaluations follow: "I liked the outward openness of all participants, having ideas tossed at you from all angles—brainstorming—to work with and improve on where *you* feel necessary. . ."; "Having contact with other women who are depressed was important to me, and realizing that others have needs such as mine. . ."; "We are helping each other outside the group, and we plan to go to school together. . ."; "I'm not the only one with problems: just because you're married doesn't mean you're happy. . ."; "I was able to obtain courage from the support in the group; I've become stronger in dealing with my problems and if it becomes necessary I can go off and live on my own without guilt. . ."; "What I learned in the group was pretty scary at times; things were brought out that I didn't like at all, and I really didn't know the feelings were inside; but—it was good for me; now it's much easier to cope with problems; I feel a lot better about myself and everyone around me; I can state my feelings without being afraid of anger. . .All in all what's really important for me is knowing I have a mouth and a brain and they both work! That makes me feel good!"

## VI. Recommendations

In addition to the subjective evaluation of the group process by the participants, the facilitators attempted to objectively measure the group members varying levels of depression. A self-report depression scale, the CES-D scale (Radloff, 1977), was administered to the group members at the initial session, after the seven semi-structured sessions, and at the closing session. As some group members chose to fill out the questionnaire at home, and failed to complete and return the questionnaires, the available data are inconclusive. Preferably, group participants would be asked to complete the questionnaires at the beginning of certain predetermined sessions to accurately measure variations in levels of depression throughout the group process.

Another suggestion is to initially plan a 10 to 16 session group; thus, more time would be allowed for the shift from a semi-structured socio-educational approach to a dynamic personal growth oriented group which requires more trust and personal openness.

Some women mentioned difficulties in making childcare arrangements. It would be advantageous to offer childcare within the agency for the period of the group sessions.

## VII. Conclusions

For many depressed women, their environments and life-styles play an intricate part in their depression; thus, the larger interpersonal and societal context must be addressed. In this 13-session group, we examined and worked on many issues in the lives of previously depressed rural women: challenging female role stereotypes, developing self-reliance rather than depending exclusively on a man, exploring and expressing anger, asserting oneself, learning to nurture oneself, and networking with each other to decrease isolation and increase female bonding and support.

Based on the positive responses of the women to this group, we believe that rural women can be assisted in decreasing their depression through a non-traditional feminist approach. Important in this process is learning to challenge societal role expectations and to develop a healthy definition of one's self. And this can be done in the supportive context of a women's group.

## REFERENCE NOTES

1. Radloff, L. S. *Sex roles, helplessness, and depression.* Unpublished Manuscript, Center for Epidemiological Studies, National Institute of Mental Health, 1978.

2. Weissman, M. M. *Depressed women: Traditional and non-traditional therapies.* Paper presented at the Eighth Annual Symposium, Effective Psychotherapy, Texas Research Institute of Mental Sciences, Houston, Texas, November 19-21, 1975.

3. Haussmann, M. J. Women's roles and vulnerability to depression (Doctoral dissertation, Western Michigan University, 1981). Dissertation Abstracts International, 1981, *42*(5), (University Microfilms No. 81-24, 216).

4. Haussmann, M. J. *Women's roles and vulnerability to depression.* Paper presented at the Eighth Annual National Conference on Feminist Psychology, Association for Women in Psychology, Boston, Massachusetts, March 5-8, 1981. (ERIC Document ED 216250)

# REFERENCES

Alper, T. Achievement motivation in college women: A now-you-see-it-now-you-don't phenomenon. In L. S. Hansen & R. S. Rapoza (Eds.), *Career development and counseling of women.* Springfield, IL: Thomas, 1978.

Arieti, S. The roots of depression: The power of the dominant other. *Psychology Today,* 1979, *12*(11), 54, 57-58, 92-93.

Beck, A. T. & Greenberg, R. L. Cognitive therapy with depressed women. In V. Franks & V. Burtle (Eds.), *Women and therapy: New psychotherapies for a changing society.* New York: Brunner/Mazel, 1974.

Bernard, J. *The future of marriage.* New York: Bantam, 1973.

Bienvenu, M. J., Sr. Inventory of anger communication. In J. W. Pfeiffer & J. E. Jones (Eds.), *The 1976 annual handbook for group facilitators.* La Jolla, CA: University Associates, 1976.

Block, J., Von der Lippe, A., & Block, J. H. Sex-role socialization patterns: Some personality concomitants and environmental antecedents. *Journal of Consulting and Clinical Psychology,* 1973, *41,* 321-341.

Brooks, L. Supermoms shift gears: Re-entry women. *The Counseling Psychologist,* 1976, *6*(2), 33-37.

Butler, P. A. *Self-assertion for women: A guide to becoming androgynous.* San Francisco: Harper & Row, 1976.

Carter, D. K. Counseling divorced women. *Personnel and Guidance Journal,* 1977, *55,* 537-541.

Fields, S. Women, poverty, depression: Blues in the red. *Innovations,* Fall 1980, pp. 2-19.

Gilbert, L. A. Feminist therapy. In A. M. Brodsky & R. T. Hare-Mustin (Eds.), *Women and psychotherapy: An assessment of research and practice.* New York: Guilford Press, 1980.

Gilmore, S. K. If you're depressed, you're probably sub-assertive. In J. R. Leppaluoto (Ed.), *Women on the move: A feminist perspective.* Eugene: University of Oregon, 1973.

Hoffman, L. W. Early childhood experiences and women's achievement motives. In M. T. S. Mednick, S. S. Tangri, & L. W. Hoffman (Eds.), *Women and achievement.* Washington, D.C.: Hemisphere, 1975.

Jakubowski, P. A. Assertive behavior and clinical problems of women. In E. I. Rawlings & D. K. Carter (Eds.), *Psychotherapy for women: Treatment toward equality.* Springfield, IL: Charles C Thomas, 1977.

Jones, J. E. & Banet, A. G., Jr. Dealing with anger. In J. W. Pfeiffer & J. E. Jones (eds.), *The 1976 annual handbook for group facilitators.* La Jolla, CA: University Associates, 1976.

Kirsh, B. Consciousness-raising groups as therapy for women. In V. Franks & V. Burtle (Eds.), *Women in therapy: New psychotherapies for a changing society.* New York: Brunner/Mazel, 1974.

Kravetz, D. F. Consciousness-raising and self-help. In A. M. Brodsky & R. T. Hare-Mustin (Eds.), *Women and psychotherapy: An assessment of research and practice.* New York: Guilford Press, 1980.

Lange, A. J. & Jakubowski, P. A. *Responsible assertive behavior: Cognitive/behavior procedures for trainers.* Champaign, IL: Research Press, 1976.

Lipman-Blumen, J. & Leavitt, H. J. Vicarious and direct achievement patterns in adulthood. In L. S. Hansen & R. S. Rapoza (Eds.), *Career development and counseling of women.* Springfield, IL: Charles C Thomas, 1978.

Manis, L., Lockwood, K., Nutter, S., Mochizuki, J., & Pattison, M. *Leader's handbook for one-day assertiveness training workshop.* Kalamazoo, MI: Susan B. Anthony Press, 1977.

Manis, L. G. & Mochizuki, J. Search for fulfillment: A program for adult women. *Personnel and Guidance Journal,* 1972, *50,* 594-599.

Messer, S. B. & Lehrer, P. M. Short-term groups with female welfare clients in a job-training program. *Professional Psychology,* 1976, *7,* 352-358.

Miller, J. G. *Toward a new psychology of women.* Boston: Beacon Press, 1976.

Pfeiffer, J. W. & Jones, J. E. *Reference guide to handbooks and annuals* (3rd ed.). La Jolla, CA: University Associates, 1979.

Radloff, L. S. Sex differences in depression: The effects of occupation and marital status. *Sex Roles,* 1975, *1,* 249-265.

Radloff, L. S. The CES-D scale: A self-report depression scale for research in the general population. *Journal of Applied Psychological Measurement,* 1977, *1,* 385-401.

Rizley, R. Depression and distortion in the attribution of causality. *Journal of Abnormal Psychology,* 1978, *87,* 32-48.

Weissman, M. M. Depression. In A. M. Brodsky & R. T. Hare-Mustin (Eds.), *Women and psychotherapy: An assessment of research and practice.* New York: Guilford Press, 1980.

Weissman, M. M. & Klerman, G. L. Sex differences and the epidemiology of depression. *Archives of General Psychiatry,* 1977, *34,* 98-111.

# The All-Women's Consciousness Raising Group as a Component of Treatment for Mental Illness

Marcelle Adolph

**ABSTRACT.** This is a description of a Women's Group in a partial hospitalization program applying a variety of group treatment modalities in the treatment of mental illness. The integration of a feminist approach to women's issues provides a supportive atmosphere conducive to change. The group experience encourages a critical evaluation of sex roles and attitudes, as well as gender and behaviors that perpetuate stereotyped roles that result in stress-producing elements in women's lifes.

The purpose of this paper is to describe the application of principles from feminist therapy and consciousness raising groups to an adult partial hospitalization program for women patients with a range of psychiatric diagnoses. The paper indicates the rationale and goals for the group, its history, its structure, and the major techniques employed.

The incidence of particular forms of mental illness is different for women than it is for men. This is because the symptoms and underlying processes for both men and women are related to gender roles, gender socialization, and life circumstances of each gender (Lewis, 1976; Gomberg & Franks, 1979). The women's group described in this paper arose from my desire to create services appropriate to women in such a setting with their unique needs and relationships to society.

---

Marcelle Adolph is a senior Psychiatric Social Worker at the Alternative Hospital Program—a partial hospitalization program of Rush-Presbyterian-St. Luke's Medical Center located in the Marshall Field IV Medical Center, 1720 W. Polk Street, Chicago, IL 60612.

*117*

Women's Consciousness Raising (CR) groups arose initially as one of the major change tools of the women's movement as a vehicle for (usually) well functioning women to use in understanding and transforming their views of themselves and other women within the larger culture. These groups provided support and education, an opportunity to practice new skills, and a chance to work for social change as well as individual change. Although the women participating in this Alternative Hospitalization Program differ in many ways from those who formed the first CR groups, they also share with all women many life issues. Frequently they, as women, perceive themselves to be like any minority group in that they share problems and feelings such as being defenseless, passive, helpless, angry, hopeless, and degraded (Kirsh, 1974).

Incorporating CR techniques in such a group was consistent with my view of the social group worker as a resource person to a group who assists members to help themselves by mediating their concerns and providing direction for addressing them. A traditional approach emphasizes interpersonal relationships within the group. A feminist approach integrates a stronger self-help emphasis and an understanding of the nature of female oppression in a sexist society (Kravetz, 1980).

## GOALS OF THE WOMEN'S GROUP

The term "feminist" is defined as a person who advocates political, social, and economic equality between women and men (Webster's New Collegiate Dictionary, 1979, p. 48). Feminist therapy incorporates an awareness of the aspects of ideology and social structure on the behavior of women with a focus on:

A. *Separating the Internal from the External.* The client learns to differentiate between what she has been taught and has accepted as socially appropriate for her from what might actually be appropriate (Gilbert, 1980).
B. *Validation of the Female Experience.* The client comes to understand the role of society in shaping all individuals and in particular, its role in shaping the behavior of women. The client learns she is not crazy (Gilbert, 1980).
C. *Exploration of Values and Attitudes by Therapists.* Therapists

constantly explore their own values and attitudes concerning women and confront tendencies within themselves towards maintaining things as they are (Gilbert, 1980).

Compared with more traditional therapies, feminist therapy also views inclusion of some topics as important to therapy with all women, e.g., rape, pregnancy, menopause, childbirth, body image, menstruation, issues of physical power and sexual preference (Gilbert, 1980).

As a feminist therapist, I felt that organizing the Women's Group as a CR group would provide a way for its members to examine issues in their own lives in terms of their social conditioning. CR groups help women understand and deal with personal problems as these are related to their sex role, conditioning and experiences with sex bias and discrimination.

The CR group, like all psychotherapies, provides supportive and confidential experiences. The major difference is in the patient-therapist relationship. Instead of an unequal and hierarchical one, it seeks peer equality among women. CR groups are based on equal sharing of resources, power, and responsibility. They are often leaderless but, for this setting, we designed a structure for the Women's Group that provided non-coercive professional leadership and intervention.

I selected the following goals and purposes to implement these principles:

1. To improve self-image and self-esteem by using assertive rather than self defeating behavior.
2. To learn the politics of oppression through active involvement in the Women's Group (such as dealing with housing problems, day care, job discrimination, public aid hassles).
3. To learn the relationship between mental illness and one's life experiences.
4. To obtain new role models through such resources as guest speakers from the Women's Movement and from famous women of all cultures through literature.
5. To explore issues that are similar for all women by de-emphasizing status roles and by including patients, students, and staff in the groups—all struggling with similar issues with some of us coping perhaps better than others.
6. To coordinate the activities and experiences of each member

of the group with interaction with her primary therapist and other treatment team members.

## GROUP SETTING, HISTORY, COMPOSITION, AND STRUCTURE

The Alternative Hospitalization Program was established in 1964 as the Adult Day Hospital by the Department of Psychiatry of Rush-Presbyterian-St. Luke's Medical Center in Chicago's West Side Medical Center Community. Patients are referred to the Alternative Hospital Program by medical staff from Rush-Presbyterian-St. Luke's medical and psychiatric in-patient units, as well as from several satellite and affiliated hospitals throughout the city. The Program provides a transition from in-patient care to return to community life whether it be work, school, family life, or volunteer work.

The Program typically serves 25 to 35 patients, two thirds of whom are women. They range in age from 16 to 76 or older, come from a wide range of socio-economic circumstances (from public aid recipients to upper middle class persons) and from various cultural and racial backgrounds. The following diagnostic categories are represented: Psychosomatic problems, stress disorders, bipolar illness, borderline disorder, severe depression, schizophrenia undifferentiated, adjustment disorders, and substance abuse. While attending the program, patients reside at home or at a sheltered facitity.

In March, 1974, I met with a handful of women for the first session on the Women's Group; the topic was "Anger." By October, 1974, eleven to twelve patients attended regularly. Students placed on the unit provided additional impetus because of their previous or current participation in women's studies. The group is now an integral part of the training program for female students in social work, nursing, occupational therapy, and medicine.

Shortly after the establishment of the Women's Group, a Men's Group was formed which meets simultaneously with the Women's Group. Four to eight male patients attend the men's group regularly. Occasionally, there are joint seesions of the Women's and Men's groups discussing issues of mutual interest. These have included such topics as "Against Female Anger," Sexuality, Women and Literature, and Women in Theology.

All female patients, staff, and students are encouraged to attend the Women's Group. Male speakers are present only at joint sessions with the Men's Group. The group has two co-therapists, myself and a staff psychiatric nurse committed to feminist issues. The group continues to attract 11-12 patients and meets weekly for one hour and 15 minutes followed by a post-group meeting to evaluate the session (with the co-therapists and students).

## PROGRAM TOPICS AND TECHNIQUES

The topics that have been addressed over the years are listed in Table 1. The topics are chosen in conjunction with each particular patient group, based on the needs and issues present in that particular group. Some topics, particularly the issues surrounding sexuality, are crucial and would not be talked about easily in a mixed setting. The co-therapists take primary responsibility for suggesting issues to be discussed based on their readings in feminist literature or featured articles in newspapers or TV programs that relate to women issues. Topics also arise at group sessions. An example is a member's reaction to stress on the job, poor pay, child care problems or sexual harassment.

Program techniques have also varied widely (see Table 2 for a listing). The most personally intense technique is the development of Herstories, described in detail later. This technique requires that the majority of the patients know and trust each other and can only work well when there has been a core of patients who have met together for a period of time—sometimes as long as two months. While working towards the development of this trust, ask the group what is most relevant for them. Often one of the patients brings an issue, topic, or article to discuss. Sometimes we are guided by a topic of incident that arose in the previous meeting or we take advantage of a topic or event that is currently receiving media attention. We have also been given information by other therapists within the program about issues that they think will be useful for their patients to discuss.

If a group is ready to initiate a discussion on some topic of their own choosing, it is usually empowering for them if this is adopted no matter how exciting the topic the leaders had prepared (assuming, of course, that the new topic is relevant and of general interest to all or most group members). Sometimes a group will not be ready

Table 1

| Program Topics<br>A Partial List of Topics Discussed in the Women's<br>Group Since Its Inception ||
|---|---|
| Title of Topic | Description of Topic |
| Anger | Toward men, mothers, social institutions, (public aid, hospitals, etc.), children, (child abuse), Black, White issues, rape. |
| Illness | Mental illness includes suicidal ideation, depression, psychosis, neurosis; physical illness means chronic and debilitating diseases, i.e., diabetes, cancer, hypertension, sickle cell anemia. |
| Health Issues | Children's diseases, emergency rooms, hospital-izations, surgery, obesity, drinking problems, women and aging, ailing parents and spouses. |
| Breaking up a Relationship | Divorce, separation, the effect on children. |
| Women and Emotions | Comparing how men handle emotions. |
| Getting Along with Women | On the job, friends, daughters, sisters, mothers mother-in-laws, grandmothers, aunts. |
| Marriage vs Careers | Marriage and love fantasies, sex and marriage, marriage vs staying single, divorce and loneliness. |
| Sexuality | Incest, masturbation, "sometimes I don't feel like having sex", douches, yeast infections, venereal disease, impotency, frigidity, homosexuality, lesbianism. |
| Attitudes Toward Work | It's a male responsibility, women should work only before marriage or until the children arrive. |

to deal with a particular task or issue even though they had expressed interest in it the week before. Thus, we have found it useful to have more than one plan for each session, as a back-up, should our first idea not be compatible with the group's needs in any given week.

Some stimulus activity or material is introduced first (outside speaker, literature, art projects or other media) followed by a discussion of the meaning and relevance of the material to the group members. Patients are encouraged to participate, but are allowed to

Table 2

| Kinds of Techniques | Description of Techniques |
|---|---|
| "Herstory" | A social history related orally by group members based on a designated outline. |
| "Women's Day" Field Trip | Movie and lunch - film seen "Women Under the Influence." Male patients furious that they were not consulted or invited. Heated debate during several community meetings. |
| Applying Several Program Media for a Specific Topic | Topic of sexuality took on a wider scope through films, speakers, and literature. Areas explored: birth control - abortion - menopause, written resources provided "How to Meet Men". |
| Providing Consultants | Attended fashion shows and provided consultants on make-up, hair styling, and fashions to group members. |
| Speakers from Feminist Organizations RE: Special Issues | Planned Parenthood Association - "Teenage Pregnancies". Church Federation of Chicago - "Housing for Women Living Alone". YWCA - "Rape - Battered Women Syndrome". |
| Photography | Sharing family life hisotry, self-identity - recalling memories. |

set their own pace and choose the form and degree of their participation in any particular session. Co-therapists participate as full members selecting experiences, thoughts and feelings to share.

Since members come and go in a setting like this, it is necessary to orient new group members in each meeting. Usually we ask one of the more experienced members to explain the group, its purposes, and how it works to new members.

## SOME REPRESENTATIVE SESSIONS

### The "Herstory"

A primary example in the Women's Group that integrates the concept of the social history into the group work process is the "Herstory" or "Her Story" (in contrast to History, or "His Story"). I designed the "Herstory" as a history that is related orally by a group member who voluntarily shares memories of "growing up female." This includes family life, school years, friendships, dating, marriage, sexual relationships, child-bearing, child-rearing and work experiences. It is an important technique in getting acquainted with "ourselves" and the forces that shape "us" (Small, 1978). A group member may take one or two entire sessions to relate her "Herstory."

This group experience can be described thusly: (1) it is a self-revelation experience and peer support provides direction, guidance, and analysis of the problems and events presented. The group centered approach de-emphasizes the role of the leader and promotes peer relationships (Kaplan, 1979). (2) One might feel frightened or anxious at the thought of exposing one's self, but actually results in a cathartic release. (3) Group involvement helps the "Herstory" teller as group members ask pertinent questions to get at unclear statements. A joint group endeavor of defining a diagnosis of the member's problems is in contrast to the dyad communication that occurs in the traditional social history work-up. (4) Each person who wishes to participate in this event is given a copy of the "Herstory Outline" a week in advance to assist her in preparing her recall of memories of her life experiences (Small, 1978). This outline is presented in Table 3. The woman is also en-

Table 3

"Herstory" Outline

To Assist Group Members' Recall

of Early and More Current Memories

of Their Life Experiences

| Questions | Clarification and Depth of Information |
|---|---|
| When and Where Were You Born? | Give explicit details if you can, which will include any knowledge of your birth and babyhood given to you by parents, siblings, relatives, and family friends. Where did you grow up? Name of town, kind of neighborhood, and size of city. |
| Describe your Parents | Include siblings and important relatives and friends. |
| Schools Years | Nursery or kindergarten - where located? Describe grammar school years - favorite teachers, subjects, and friends. With high school, do same as above and include extra curricular activities. Do the same if your attended college. |
| Work History | First job, current employment, other jobs. |
| Dating | Describe your first date. |
| Menstruation | When did you first menstruate? How old were you? Where did it occur? How prepared were you? Who gave you information? Mother, father, sister, girlfriend, or relative. |
| Sex Information | Who told you how babies were made? Who taught you about sex? Do you think you have enough information or knowledge about sex, birth control? |

Table 3, continued.

| Pregnancy | What, where, when and from whom did you learn about child-rearing? What was your first pregnancy like? |
|---|---|
| Decisions | What was the most important decision you ever made? What was the most important event in your life? What are your goals? |
| Family History | Is there history of family violence, i.e., sexual abuse, emotional abuse, physical abuse? |

couraged to bring family memorabilia, photos, or other materials to illustrate her discussion.

The following examples illustrate how CR group support and empathy can facilitate a woman's developing a new understanding of her life and her options through a sharing of her "Herstory."

*Case I:* Mary, 50 years old, separated from husband. Diagnosis: Neurotic Depression. Mary was very depressed when she entered the group. In relating her "Herstory," she came to the following episode: Her husband was very drunk, beat her severely and then threw her out of the window from their second floor apartment. She was hospitalized for almost a year. As she related this crisis in her life, she became very agitated.

It appeared that she had never related this event in treatment sessions. Her primary therapist saw her immediately following the group session to deal with this issue. Her depression lifted in a few weeks and she was able to eventually return to work.

*Case II:* Helene, 60 years old, widow. Diagnosis: Manic Depressive Illness including a multitude of somatic complaints, Helene had been a professional actress doing monologues throughout the United States during her younger years. She felt depleted, alone, isolated, impoverished, living on Public Aid, when in the past, she had been married to a physician and lived in comparative luxury. Helen's "Herstory" was an exciting oral document presented as a dramatic musical event like her former theatrical monologues. She was enthusiastically applauded by the group and encouraged to resume her theatrical life by entertaining senior citizen groups. Helene seemed pleased with that suggestion and did follow through following discharge from the Alternative Hospital Program.

## THE USE OF READING MATERIAL

One technique that works well is to introduce literature for discussion by providing multiple copies so that members take turns reading aloud, followed by group discussion. Introducing a topic that is pertinent to an all women group and discussing it in a non-clinical manner, can generate meaningful, but non-threatening discussions that often lead the group into deeper levels of sharing and self-disclosure. Women who are miles apart socially, culturally, ethnically, and economically often discover that they had similar experiences. Such discoveries help the women identify how being women has affected their experiences and tends to decrease the self-criticism and self-blame that many women have.

In one session, the therapist knew that several members were working on mother-daughter relationships. By sharing with the group an Ann Landers column (a source well known and respected by group members), she generated a discussion of how families deal with secrets as well as of issues related to poor mother-daughter communication and lack of appropriate nurturing.

The letter described a daughter's lament that she had never appreciated or understood her mother's concern for her; only after her death did she realize what a loss it was to her that she and her mother could never come to grips with their unhappy relationship.

One member was currently in the throes of a hostile-dependent relationship with a critically ill and hospitalized mother, who refused to see her daughter (patient) but later allowed her to visit her briefly. The mother told her she never wanted to see her again. The patient described how her mother abused her physically as a child, and later in adult life, had her committed to a mental institution and placed her children in foster care.

The group was exposed to this patient's pain, and the members expressed their concern and support so that this woman could feel supported and come to trust the group members.

Within this session, another 22-year-old member related an incident that occurred when she was 17 years old. She had an abortion by a physician who depreciated her fears and pain. Fortunately she was accompanied by a friend who took care of her following the abortion. The young woman was unable to relate this crucial incident until recently to her mother, a former nurse, or to her father, a prominent physician. She felt safe enough to share this frightening experience outside the family unit.

She had difficulty tolerating the positive feedback that she had made a decision (the abortion) that was to her advantage and welfare, and has always been ambivalent about any independent decisions. She had expected criticism from the group. This patient also felt obligated to her family to keep secrets and accept the attitudes of doctors. "After all, I am the daughter of a doctor," she said.

There was some discussion of the similar feelings experienced by both of these very different women about their families, especially their mothers. The group process and the facilitators are beginning to fill in some of the nurturing gaps so that the members can begin to work on nurturing themselves.

## USE OF THERAPIST ROLE MODELING

The inner feelings and thoughts of the co-therapists are not unlike our patients. In many sessions, when we think it will be helpful to the group members to recognize this, we discuss with each other and the group some of our own experiences, thoughts, and feelings. The patients usually listen with much interest when we do this. When we seemed less different from them, this decreased the status gap between staff and patients.

Some of the kinds of thoughts we shared with the group were that we also experience male therapists as depreciating women, male doctors as not "having time" for their female patients, and how the women's movement has influenced us. We also expressed our perceptions as to how gender factors affect other professions in the hospital such as the way doctors and nurses relate to each other—the doctors issuing orders to the nurses.

## USE OF MUSIC AND ART

At one session when the men's group and women's group were together we used music to stimulate interaction. We played Ravel's *Bolero* and asked the patients to write a story stimulated by the music.

All of the women patients related stories about princesses being rescued by ardent suitors (all princes, of course) and being rewarded by marriage to these princesses. The princes performed deeds of heroism and won many battles.

The stories created by the men told of the heroic and daring deeds that men do such as saving the life of a princess and then being offered the reward of the princess in marriage. Only one male patient related a story about himself. He was out with his wife and children on a ride in the country to have a picnic. All was peaceful and lovely. In reality, this man's marriage was collapsing and he isolates himself from his wife and children. He denies the reality of his situation and attempts to be in power through fantasy, wishes for the way it used to be when he was the breadwinner. His wife is now working.

The men's stories depicted adventure, conquest, and power. The women depicted themselves as passive, waiting to be rescued from their unhappiness. We wonder what the content of their stories would be like if they had met separately.

## COORDINATION AND BETWEEN-SESSION WORK

It is very important that the co-therapists of such a group stay in regular communication with the patients' primary therapists. The therapist can be very helpful in identifying issues that would be productive to discuss in the group, and should be alerted to follow-up on topics and content that emerges in the group. Also, the therapists may want to assign "homework" (like the "Herstory" preparation) or follow-up with a patient after the group session.

For instance, in the session described earlier with the discussions of marriage, one member in this session was silent throughout the hour. Because of an organic illness, the woman is losing her vision, hearing, and sense of touch. One is never sure if she is listening because of her bland affect. After this session, I approached her and asked her how she felt about this topic of marriage. She is a widow, dependent on relatives to care for her, whereas, in the past, she had been an active, hardworking woman.

She responded by describing her husband—an alcoholic who physically abused her. She said in a loud, angry tone that she was glad he was dead. I asked her if she was willing to share this at the next session of the Women's Group. She agreed to do so and verbalized her pain and anger that she kept hidden under her stoic appearance at the next session.

## CONCLUDING REMARKS

This article illustrates ways that feminist principles and CR techniques can be applied in an all-women group in a day hospital program. The women's group has been an enormously helpful component of treatment for those who have participated in it.

Most of the female patients have led isolated lives and this is the first time they have joined together with other women to problem-solve and to say what they can't say anywhere else. The similarity and commonality of women's lives shared in this kind of group breaks down their isolation and frees its members to consider alternatives rather than hold on to devalued personality traits, attitudes and behaviors.

We as therapists continue to be alerted to our own needs as we focus on our patients' needs. And so we continue to explore new feminist literature and seminars and stay active in our own Women's Organizations. To organize and run such a group requires a firm commitment to feminist philosophy, and an understanding of gender and its effects on personality development and socialization of women in our society.

## RESOURCE BIBLIOGRAPHY

Brownmiller, S. *Against Our Will, Men, Women and Rape.* New York: Simon & Schuster, 1975.

Chester, P. *Women and Madness.* New York: Avon Books, 1972.

Churchill, R. S. and Glasser, N. R. Small groups in the mental hospital. In: P. Glasser, R. Sarri, R. Vinter (Eds.). *Individual Change Through Small Groups.* New York: Free Press, 1974.

Ebrenreich, B. and English, D. *Witches, Midwives, and Nurses: A History of Women Healers.* Glass Mountain Pamphlet, No. 1, New York: Feminist Press, 1973.

Gerth, N. and Mills, C. W. *Character and Social Structure.* New York: Harcourt, Brace and Worls, 1953.

Greer, G. *The Female Eunuch.* New York: McGraw-Hill Book Co., 1971.

Millet, K. *Sexual Politics.* New York: Doubleday and Co., Inc., 1970.

Morgan, R. (Ed.). *Sisterhood is Powerful: An Anthology of Writings from The Women's Liberation Movement.* New York: Vintage Books, 1970.

*Ms. Magazine.* New York: Ms. Foundation for Education and Communication Inc.

*National New Times.* Official Journal of the National Organization for Women (NOW).

Polk, B. B. and Stein, R. B. Is the grass greener on the other side? In: C. Safilios-Rothchild (Ed.). *Toward a sociology of women.* Lexington, Mass. Xerox, 1972.

# REFERENCES

Brodsky, A. M. and Hare-Mustin, R. (Eds.). *Women and Psychotherapy: An assessment of research and practice.* New York: The Guilford Press, 1980.

Brown, M. A. and Rodolfo, A. Chicanos and social group work models: Some implications for group work practice. *Social Work with Groups,* 1979, *4,* 331-341.

Feminists issue call to action; Ask Professional to take lead role. *N.A.S.W. News,* Nov., 1979, 25.

Frank, J. The bewildering world of psychotherapy. *Journal of Social Issues,* 1972, *28,* 27-44.

Franks, V. and Burtle, V. (Eds.). *Women in Psychotherapy: New psychotherapies for a Changing Society.* New York: Brunner/Mazel, 1974.

Gilbert, L. A. Feminist therapy. In A. M. Brodsky and R. Hare-Mustin (Eds.). *Women and Psychotherapy: An Assessment of Research and Practice.* New York: The Guilford Press, 1980.

Gomberg, E. and Franks, V. (Eds.). *Gender and Disordered Behavior: Sex Differences in Psychopathology.* New York: Brunner/Mazel, 1979.

Kaplan, I. H. Clinical work with individuals and groups. *Social Work with Groups,* 1979, *4,* pp. 295-307.

Kirsh, B. Consciousness raising groups as therapy for women. In B. Franks and V. Burtle (Eds.). *Women in Therapy: New Psychotherapies for a Changing Society.* New York: Brunner/Mazel, 1974.

Kravetz, D. Consciousness raising and self help. In A. M. Brodsky and R. Hare-Mustin (Eds.). *Women and Psychotherapy: An Assessment of Research and Practice.* New York: The Guilford Press, 1980.

Levine, B. *Fundamentals of Group Treatment.* Chicago: Whitehall Co., 1967.

Lewis, H. B. *Psychic War in Women and Men.* New York: New York University Press, 1976.

Small, S. M. *Outline for Psychiatric Examination.* East Hanover, N.J. Sandoz Pharmaceuticals Pamphlet, 71978.

*Webster's New Collegiate Dictionary.* Springfield, Mass.: Merriman, 1979.

# A Self-Help Group for Women in Abusive Relationships

## Susan Hartman

**ABSTRACT.** Some innovative aspects of an ongoing group for women in violent relationships are discussed. The philosophical framework includes a broad definition of violence and a focus on empowerment of women. The self-help group model which provides the form for this group offers special features: minimal entry requirements, options in style of participation, and dual leadership with both a lay and professional person. Predictable phases of participants' focus which are described include: self-esteem, self-protection, catharsis, autonomy and support, and issues related to patterns of violence. The author believes that the philosophy, self-help group form, and permission for a wide range of focus in this group are particularly suited to meet the needs of women in abusive relationships.

This paper will describe the therapeutic self-help group for women in abusive relationships. This weekly group has open membership, with an average attendance of nine women. Fifty-eight women were served in the first seventeen months of the group. Twenty came to one or two sessions only. Nine members have been part of the group for ten to seventeen months. The average length of stay in the group is approximately four months.

## PHILOSOPHY OF SERVICE

The present name of the group, "Self-Help Group for Women in Abusive Relationships," evolved over the first weeks of the group. At its inception the group, like many others in the community, was

Susan Hartman is counselor and family life educator at Family and Children's Service, 414 South Eighth Street, Minneapolis, MN 55404.

This paper is a revision of a presentation at the Regional Women's Conference of the National Association of Social Workers, Minneapolis, Minnesota in May, 1982.

The author thanks Jane Hynes, Carole Mae Olson, and Ted Bowman for their support and suggestions.

*133*

labeled "Group for Battered Women." Other names seemed un-wieldly. However two conclusions grew out of observations of the women's work and led to a change of the name and of the philosoph-ical underpinnings of this group.

First, I recognized that labeling women in violent relationships, who already feel helpless and dependent, as "battered women" fostered their victimization stance. Indeed, women are battered and are victims. Repeatedly acknowledging these facts to the women is imperative. Working with the women as part of an abusive system, however, can both encourage this awareness and also support a focus on the women's strengths and on the importance of their tak-ing responsibility for their lives.

Then, as I listened to the reports of the women, I realized that some of the women were themselves abusive. Often the women abused in reaction to the violence of their partner; sometimes they initiated the abuse, acting out patterns they learned in their families of origin. Regardless of how or why the women were abusive, their own violence created difficulties for them. Labeling the women "battered women" made it too easy to avoid confronting the mem-bers' abusive patterns.

The name of the group and the concomitant philosophical stance fits with five basic tenets about violence which are the backbone of our treatment approach.

First, violence is not acceptable. The only possible exception is self-defense.

Second, "Violent family members are not to blame for having this problem. . . . There is a hurt child within the attacking adult and the victim does not cause the attack" (Cantoni, 1981, p. 8). No one deserves or is responsible for another's violence. Yet while abuse is not the result of the relationship, it is destructive to both part-ners in it.

Third, "Each member of a violent family must assume respon-sibility for change. No one outside the family can bestow peace. . ." (Cantoni, 1981, p. 8).

Fourth, any one of four forms of destructive behavior contribute to an abusive relationship. One incident of physical violence creates such a relationship and often removes restraints against further violence (Shainess, 1977). The other three types of abuse—sexual violence, destruction of property dear to one's partner, and psycho-logical/verbal abuse—can result from and/or lead to physical violence. A relationship is not abuse free until all forms of violence cease.

Fifth, abuse can stop. Violence is learned. Violent behavior is not viewed as a natural, instinctive response. Except in very rare instances, a physical illness is not responsible for violence. A person's family of origin, cultural stereotypes, social violence, random reinforcement, and/or knowledge deficits can teach violent behavior or expectation of violence (Strauss, 1977). Because violence and the anticipation of it are learned behaviors, they can be unlearned and new behaviors learned.

Given these five beliefs, the goals for work with women in abusive relationships became fostering autonomy, a sense of empowerment and responsibility, a mastery over the environment, and improved self-image. The philosophy of the group, symbolized by the name, and the form of the group described below support these goals.

## THE SELF-HELP GROUP

The resocialization of women in abusive relationships can be accomplished within a group setting with particular effectiveness. The specific form of group chosen is the self-help model. The reasons that a group approach in general and a self-help mode in specific are appropriate for this population are enumerated below.

A group as a method of treatment provides "curative factors" (Yalom, 1975) which aid women in abusive relationships in four ways. First, the act of joining a group immediately breaks the isolation that is typical of this population. Second, by merely attending a group for women in abusive relationships—much less verbally acknowledging their condition within the first or second meeting— the women divulge their long-kept secret: they are in violent relationships. Third, hope and trust are experienced as this secret is shared, not with a therapist but with a group of persons who have had the same experience and are successfully dealing with their problems. Fourth, a group mode allows members to participate in many ways: by listening, observing, talking about their own problems, or relating to and helping others. Though this experience is intense, the women can choose how they use the group. Permission to have this choice is empowering for women who may never have had a disclosing or trusting relationship. A one-to-one therapy experience may also prove to be too intense for some clients.

The self-help model, sometimes called the mutual help system, (Golan, 1981) provides the specific form for this group. Several ingredients characterize the self-help nature of this group and make it particularly appropriate to women in abusive relationships.

## Entry Requirements

Women must currently be or previously have been in abusive relationships, and they must want to work on these and related issues. Once they have been referred to the group—generally by a counselor, an agency, or the court system—they first call either the professional or lay leader to hear how the group operates. They then attend the sessions without registration, payment, or a contract for any number of sessions. The women are encouraged to come to at least four meetings and to call a group member or the leaders to indicate that they are safe if they cannot attend a meeting. The only rigid group rules are confidentiality, no violence, and no use of chemicals before the group. The group is open-ended, and available to old and new members at any time. These minimal entrance requirements are important for this population who often feel unable to make a more substantial commitment given their chaotic lives, low self-esteem, and intense shame.

## Peer Support

"The group emphasizes the power of the members to assist one another, rather than depend on the help of professionals" (Olson & Shapiro, 1979, p. 13). The members first observe others who are further along in the learning process. They can identify with that person for hope and information. Over time, they become the more experienced members who affirm and teach new members (Silverman, 1978).

During this process the group provides a constant reality check. The women's denial and skewed perceptions about what behavior is abusive are quickly challenged by other group members. Likewise, as members interact in the group, they modify misinformation that may have arisen out of socialization deficits and/or isolation regarding roles, child rearing techniques, expression of feelings, and personal rights. Many of the members have never perceived females as powerful or competent. As they build respect for other women, the members increase their self-respect.

## Member Ownership

A self-help group clearly belongs to the members. The agency provides supportive services—a monthly list of names and phone numbers, a meeting location, advocacy services, and the expertise of a professional—rather than intrusive services. The women work together as peers rather than as dependents on authority figures. The self-help process combats learned helplessness by empowering its members. Members are encouraged to seek service and support from other sources as well.

## Dual Leadership

A professional and sponsor (myself), and an indigenous leader (the chairperson) have responsibility for this program. Both of us attend all group meetings.

The chairperson, a woman who is herself working out issues from a history of abusive relationships, leads the meetings and serves as the key contact person for the members during the week. The chairperson was not selected by me. She volunteered for this job at the beginning of the group. She had no prior leadership training. She had barely begun dealing with her violent relationship. Her motives for performing this role included a desire to help others, increase her own skills, and learn more about abusive relationships.

The chairperson's tasks include starting each session, stating the rules of the group, asking which members want to work, and focusing the discussion. She also retains her role as a member, using the group just as any other member does, by allowing the sponsor to take over the leadership functions when she works on personal issues. Because the chairperson bridges the roles of leader and member, she effectively serves as a model for other members. A hierarchical system, with which the women are all too familiar, is thus largely eliminated in the self-help model.

My job as the professional sponsor has many roles. The sponsor's tasks complement and support the chairperson's main leadership role (Holmes, 1978). Specifically, I serve as a second role model, one who stands outside the system of the chairperson and members. I display alternatives to the members' own patterns by being powerful without being abusive, tender without being abused, assertive without being aggressive, appreciative of men without being dependent, autonomous without being isolated, and surely how to be imperfect without losing self-esteem.

While the above modeling is indirect, many aspects of my tasks as therapist, educator, and advocate are more apparent. As the expert on group dynamics, I back up the chairperson as needed by clarifying process and providing behavioral options. An example of this occurred when several long-term group members demanded that a new member express her feelings rather than discuss her thoughts. Observing the rush of speech and the fragile stance of the new member, I noted to the group the important first step of acknowledging one's situation and reminded the members how difficult it had been for them to share their feelings at first. Another example of the need for sponsor intervention took place when one group member stopped another from relating her own experiences during a third member's work time. I discussed the varied ways of learning and growing, noting that some people learn best by relating to others rather than having the focus on themselves. A third example took place when a woman venting her anger crossed the line to abusiveness of another member by name-calling. I labeled this behavior abusive, said this would not be allowed in the group, and aided the chairperson to help members examine this interaction.

What I do as sponsor within the meetings is only part of my job. My activities outside the meetings include publicizing the group, taking referrals, interacting with referral sources, acting as liaison with the members' individual counselors, and handling crises that occur between meetings (e.g., helping members obtain legal protection or encouraging them to report child abuse). The expectation that is slowly being realized is that the chairperson and group members will take over many of these responsibilities.

Of great importance is my on-going support to the chairperson. The chairperson-sponsor relationship is a delicate and powerful one and is critical to the life of the group. This particular relationship has changed over the course of the group. At first, the weekly meetings of the two leaders consisted largely of my supporting her personal growth and teaching her about group process and abuse. As she increased her leadership skills and moved away from her own abusive relationships, the sessions between us were focused more on particular problems within the group. The relationship eased along a continuum from a therapist-client, teacher-student model toward a collaborative undertaking with mutual support, teaching, and planning. The chairperson has now completed a leadership training program and has begun college work toward a degree in the social sciences.

## Issues in the Sponsor Role

Potentially dangerous situations inside and outside the group sessions offer a challenge. Danger to the sponsor is a possibility, and dangerous situations with group members and their partners are a reality. New rules about walking to cars in groups have been necessary because some members' partners have threatened them after the group meetings.

Another risk to the sponsor is in forgetting that both partners in abusive relationships are humans in pain who have learned negative behavior patterns and are themselves victims. Margaret Elbow notes that

> it is important that the helping person not berate the abuser either directly or by innuendo. . . . If the victim senses that the counselor sees her husband as one without any positive qualities, she may become defensive of him. . . . Without recognition of her ambivalence, she feels alienated, not only from her husband, friends, and family but also from her counselor. (1977, p. 524)

Leading an education group for men and women in abusive relationships has allowed me to maintain a sense of perspective. I have had the opportunity to listen to the partners of some of the women in the self-help group talk about their own pasts, concerns, and hopes. This experience has tempered my disapproval of the men's behavior with a sense of compassion.

A sponsor's attitude toward the women themselves can easily become one of frustration, with swings from distancing to countertransference.

> practitioners may respond with disbelief, blame, or even hostility towards the victim. . .Or, the helplessness and dependence of the battered woman can result in the clinician taking inappropriate responsibility for the victim rather than helping her to become a more autonomous person capable of assuming responsibility for herself. (King, 1981, p. 8)

By being open to learning from the members as well as teaching them and by encouraging members to help each other in appropriate self-help style, I have attempted to maintain a healthy distance rather than over-involvement or total detachment. Working with this group can be draining both emotionally and physically and it has been important for me, in the agency and the community, to have a support system.

## PHASES OF WORK

The phases through which each woman moves as she works in the group are complex yet predictable. From observation, I have come to identify six stages: self-focus, self-worth, development of a protection plan, catharsis, autonomy and support, and work on issues related to violence. With each new phase comes deeper levels of examination.

### Phase One: Self-Focus

In spite of the pre-group information which stresses that members must work on their own issues, most women enter this support group believing they will learn ways to change their abusive partners. In order to make use of the group, these women must begin to focus on themselves. When new members attend the group, more experienced group members help them toward a self-focus with questions such as "But what were your feelings?" or "What do *you* want to do?" Relating incidents of abuse is both encouraged and allowed and can be done within this stage. Self-focus cannot be over-emphasized. Talking about one's partner is non-productive. Autonomy and a sense of powerfulness begins when a woman is willing to examine her own issues, choices, feelings, and behavior. This often represents a change in life-long patterns of other-directedness and dependence.

### Phase Two: Self-Worth

The second phase of work which the members must move through was not apparent to me for some months. It gradually became evident that many women were unable to develop plans to protect themselves. What was holding them back was their lack of belief that they did not deserve to be abused. Some women have never known any relationships that were not violent and have no awareness that anything else is possible. Others have low self-esteem. Still other women's depression prevents them from recognizing their own rights and worth. Experienced group members challenge the perceptions, validate the strengths, and offer unconditional acceptance—though not always approval—to newer members. As a result, these members build self-esteem and gain a clearer sense of their rights. Without some basic belief in their worth and capabilities, women will not develop plans to protect themselves from violence. If they manage to build a protection plan but lose a sense of self-worth, they often return to an estranged partner and/or leave the group.

## Phase Three: Development of a Protection Plan

Developing a protection plan was originally viewed as the first order of business for women in the group. A protection plan is an individual's unique, pre-determined behavioral approach to dealing with a partner's abuse. Formulating this plan requires the women to understand many aspects of violence, know how the courts and police can assist, and be aware of their partner's specific patterns as well as their own. Each woman must understand the cycle of violence: the cues of the buildup, the explosion, and the honeymoon stages. Then she must personalize this awareness by examining previous episodes of violence to discover the cues that indicate abuse is approaching. These cues might be a look on the partner's face, behavior such as drinking or coerced sex, a period of time since the last violence, or internal cues such as fear or anxiety. Most women will first discover cues close to the explosion point. The group urges them to look for cues which are minutes or days earlier in their partner's particular cycle of violence.

Once aware of cues, women must decide how they will protect themselves when the signals occur. They may, for instance, obtain a legal restraining order, call the police, leave the house, move to another room, go to a shelter, have a friend come over, or ask for a "time out." Women with children include them in their plans, sometimes keeping keys, money, and clothing in a diaper bag.

Some women who do have the necessary self-esteem remain unable to formulate protection plans. Five reasons for this problem are evident. First, women's situations may be so dangerous that they need immediate legal protection to ensure their safety. In such cases, members are encouraged to and sometimes aided in the process of obtaining restraining orders or filing assault charges.

A second reason for the inability to develop a protection plan is a fear of being abandoned with insufficient economic resources. A third reason can be women's confusion about what is, in fact, abusive. Forced sex, hiding of car keys, and ripping out the phone typify behaviors which some women fail to identify as abusive and as cues of personal harm to come.

Chemical abuse is a fourth reason some women are unable to protect themselves. Referrals for assessment and treatment are made in such instances. I believe that most women cannot successfully protect themselves when they are chemically dependent. This in no way implies that women's drug use is an excuse for or a cause of their partner's violence.

A fifth reason, though unusual, for failure to form safety plans is the woman's own violence. Women who themselves name-call, coerce or hit other than in self-defense often need to work on halting their own violence while also protecting themselves from their partner's abuse. In such situations action plans are developed to deal with prevention of abuse by *oneself*—searching for cues of rising anger and violence within oneself and then making specific plans to stop oneself from being abusive. While the need for women to work on their own abuse before formulating safety plans is rare, most women, in the course of their stay in the group, discover some behavior patterns which they define as abusive and wish to modify through an action plan.

### Phase Four: Catharsis

The fourth stage of work that the women move through is venting. Expression of emotions and recounting of experiences take place through all stages of a woman's work. As has been noted, the sharing of the secret of being in an abusive relationship happens early in a person's work. Spewing out this information and being accepted in spite of it reduces shame and allows the women to focus on themselves in Phase One. However, a more intense period of catharsis seems to take place once a workable protection plan is completed and the physical violence has ceased.

Any or all of the women's feelings might be discharged at this stage. These include responses to the violence (terror, panic, depression, lack of control) or affects stemming from earlier family-of-origin deprivation. Often women in this phase see no end to their feelings of loss and emptiness. They sometimes ask to be held during the meetings. The group becomes a safe place, a haven in which members can receive nurturing and controls as they constructively vent their feelings.

## Phase Five: Autonomy and Support

The fear that often replaces the sadness and anger leads to this phase, work on autonomy issues and simultaneous development of support systems. The women learn the difference between symbiotic, co-dependent relationships and autonomous, interdependent interchanges. Assertiveness skills are often a focus at this stage as the members begin to understand the distinction between abuse and limit setting, caretaking and caring about, and selfishness and self-respect. A member needs a great deal of strength, new information, support, and confronting to believe, for instance, that she is not a bad, selfish person for wanting some time without her partner or children and to be with friends of her own choosing.

Work on developing autonomous behavior is a step beyond work on changing perceptions about autonomy. Often the behavioral changes take place within the group itself. Women's passive roles and actions are challenged. Women who allow themselves to be victims in the group are taught assertiveness skills. Still other women who become aggressive and abusive as they struggle with independence issues are given controls. New behaviors can then be transferred to relationships outside the group.

As the members develop a sense of autonomy, they begin to gather and use support systems. Besides joining other groups, the members learn to turn to each other between group sessions. Frequently the group will contract for one member to either initiate or receive phone calls from other members. Some members report that this is the first time in their lives they have had friendships. The new support sometimes takes pressure off primary relationships and enables women to undertake risk-laden activities such as job training. Without some support, a member has difficulty maintaining self-esteem and autonomy.

Women who have worked through the above issues often subtly make a decision at this point. They focus either on themselves or on their relationship. While working on one's relationship or focusing on oneself are not mutually exclusive choices, members do appear to concentrate on one more than the other. Some members seek couple counseling and/or move back to an estranged partner. These women are encouraged to remain in the group. Other women develop new relationships. Some women have affairs. The group neither condones nor disapproves of the affairs outright, but helps members look at their motives, feelings, and behaviors.

Some women stall in their progress during this phase because of fear of either dependence or independence. Often members become obsessive about, for example, their feelings of shame, anger or sadness, about their history, their partners, or about men in general. Though the concerns are generally valid, the obsession itself serves as a defense against dealing with the women's own neediness and emptiness.

Hysteria provides another unconscious stall tactic which is common in the group. Some members dwell in a dramatic way on crisis after crisis. In the process, these women defend against their fear of autonomy and independence. Once these patterns of obsession or hysteria become apparent, members are confronted. For willing group members, I offer referrals for individual counseling.

## Phase Six: Related Issues

After the phase on autonomy, work takes place that is not so clearly demarcated. Long term group members continue their work on issues of self-focus, self-worth, protection, venting, autonomy and support by applying them to areas of their life that have been affected by or do affect their involvement in abusive relationships. Sexuality, communication styles, work-related issues, friendships, family of origin patterns, shame, incest, and child rearing issues concern nearly all the women.

Moving through the six phases has taken many months for the first members of this self-help group. Now, as newer members are exposed early in their involvement in the group to the current work of long-term members, the former begin to integrate the issues of Phase Six into their earlier work. It remains unclear what impact, if any, this new integration of work stages will have.

With the exception of the protection plan, these steps are in no way structured into a member's work by the leaders. No woman masters all the areas mentioned above. Members may choose to leave during any one of the stages. Each member assesses her growth and determines what support systems she can use in the future before departing from the group, although she is always welcome to return.

## CONCLUDING REMARKS

Several aspects of this particular self-help group may seem disturbing to traditional group workers. The relationship of the chairperson and sponsor forms the backbone of the group and will vary depending on the strengths and skills of the lay leader. Though the woman who offers to be chairperson need not be the strongest group member, the self-selection process generally yields a woman who can learn. The absence of entry requirements and contract for time commitment to the group suports rather than repels the women's involvement. I emphasize that the group, its leaders, and its philosophy continue to evolve.

A comment from a member after attending her first session and notes from a woman in Phase Six speak, finally, of the impact of this group on the women in abusive relationships.

Now I know I am loved and understood. (first time member)

Originally I found comfort in being with other women like me. I had felt so alone before. Now I believe I have a family. I have found acceptance, love, a consistant support of who I am. I have really grown. I have begun to heal. The group has given me the skills to begin again. The support I have found there has been the foundation for me. My life would not be as it is today without my group. (member of one year)

## REFERENCES

Cantoni, L. Clinical issues in domestic violence. *Social Casework*, 1981, *62*, 3-12.

Elbow, M. Theoretical considerations of violent marriages. *Social Casework*, 1977, *58*, 515-526.

Golan, N. *Passing Through Transitions: A Guide for Practioners.* New York: The Free Press, 1981.

Holmes. S. Parents anonymous: A treatment method for child abuse. *Social Work*, 1978, *23*, 245-247.

King, L. S. Responding to spouse abuse: The mental health profession. *Response*, Newsletter for Center for Women Policy Studies, May/June, 1981, 6-9.

Olson, C. M. and Shapiro, M. A combined therapeutic and self-help approach in working with former and current prostitutes. Unpublished paper, Minneapolis, 1979.

Shainess, N. Psychological aspects of wifebeating. In Roy, M (ed.) *Battered Women: A Psychological Study of Domestic Violence.* New York: Van Nostrand Reinhold Co., 1977.

Silverman, P. R. Mutual help: An alternate network. In *Women in Mid-life Security and Fulfillment.* Select Committee on Aging, U.S. House of Representatives, Washington, D.C.: U.S. Government Printing Office, 1978.

Star, B. et al. Psychological aspects of wife battering. *Social Casework,* 1979, *60,* 479-487.

Strauss, M. A sociological perspective on the prevention and treatment of wifebeating. In Roy, M. (ed.) *Battered Women: A Psychological Study of Domestic Violence.* New York: Van Nostrand Reinhold Co., 1977.

Yalom, I. D. *The Theory and Practice of Group Psychotherapy.* New York: Basic Books, Inc., 1975.

# PRACTICE WITH MEN

# An Overview of Men's Groups

Terry S. Stein

**ABSTRACT.** Men's groups have existed for a variety of purposes, including consciousness-raising, support, education, counseling, and psychotherapy, for several years, but they have been described infrequently in the literature. This overview of men's groups presents a rationale for such groups in terms of changing perspectives on the masculine gender role. It also describes several applications for two specific types of men's groups, consciousness-raising and psychotherapy groups. The author discusses some of his own experiences as a leader in men's groups as well. The author states that the future of men's groups depends on an increased use of these groups and on more extensive reporting about them in the professional literature.

Groups of men have existed throughout history. Most of these groups, whether large in size, such as an all male army or religious order, or small, such as a meeting of the male tribal leaders in a primitive society or a gathering of a totally male corporate board of directors in an industrial society, have both reflected and served to maintain cultural definitions of masculine and feminine gender roles. Men have met in these all male groups to perform certain functions which have most often been separated from the functions women perform. The purpose of this article is to discuss a type of men's group which differs from these other exclusively male groups. The specific functions of this type of men's group are to encourage examination of how the masculine gender role is experienced by individual men and to explore new ways of enacting this role.

Several types of such men's groups can be described based upon the stated purposes and the format of the group. These include support, political action, consciousness-raising, discussion, education, counseling, and psychotherapy groups. All of these types of men's

Terry S. Stein is Associate Professor in Psychiatry and Director of Medical Student Programs in Psychiatry, Department of Psychiatry, College of Osteopathic Medicine and College of Human Medicine, Michigan State University, East Lansing, MI 48824.

*149*

groups share two characteristics: (1) at some point in their life they are all male in composition, and (2) during the course of the group an opportunity is provided to discuss or take action regarding concerns related to the masculine gender role. Only two major categories of such men's groups, consciousness-raising groups and counseling or psychotherapy groups, are described in this article.

The history of men's groups in America is short and poorly documented, but demonstrates several important issues. First, while a few published references exist, actual studies have been practically nonexistent until recently. Second, the phenomenon of men's groups came after the start of the women's movement and the formation of a large number of women's groups. Third, the history of men's groups reflects some of the problems inherent in all male groups. These problems include the difficulty for a group of men who themselves represent masculinity to accomplish the task of "unbecoming" men* and the related difficulty of developing strategies for groups which are not stereotypically masculine but which will at the same time allow honest expression of the masculinity of the group's members.

## RATIONALE FOR MEN'S GROUPS

The fundamental rationale for men's groups is a belief in the need for men as a group to change their behaviors, belief systems and affective experiences. A number of authors have discussed the problems for men in these areas (Farrell, 1974a; Fasteau, 1974; Goldberg, 1976; Pleck & Pleck, 1980; Tolson, 1977). I have identified sex specific areas of concern for men related to gender role issues: a generalized difficulty and anxiety in related to the changing role of women in society, changes in the fathering role, examination of the male role in work and recreation, a wish by men to change affective style, alterations in the nature of adult relationships, and changing patterns of sexual functioning (Stein, 1979).

From my own work with several men's groups and from the few descriptions of men's groups in the literature (Farrell, 1974b; Moreland, 1976; Washington, 1979; Wong, 1978), a list of purposes and functions of men's groups can be derived. Such a rationale serves to

---

*"Unbecoming men" is a term derived from the title of the first published report about a men's groups which described the experiences of the men in a men's consciousness-raising group (Bradley et al., 1971).

differentiate men's groups from other types of groups and to describe the unique contributions of men's groups to society in general and to counseling and psychotherapy in particular. These purposes are the following:

1. Participation in a men's group itself represents a statement of non-traditional masculine values and allows men who wish to change themselves as men to begin this process by affiliating with a group of other men who have similar values and interests.
2. Men's groups provide an opportunity for men to relate to other men in an interpersonal setting without women. In such a setting, men may learn to perform many functions, such as nurturing and caretaking, which they often feel can only be done by women.
3. Men's groups serve as a means for demonstrating to men how they behave when they are with other men. The masculine-associated characteristics, such as competitiveness, aggression, and independence, can be expected to appear in groups of men meeting together, and in time men in men's groups may learn to express these characteristics in new ways.
4. The relationships in a men's group can serve to highlight the ways in which members have related to other significant men in their lives. If the group facilitates the experiencing and sharing of the "here and now" male-male relationships, its members may acquire a greater understanding of the ways in which they, both as individual men and men in groups, are encouraged to interact with other men according to stereotyped masculine patterns.
5. A men's group can provide a setting in which to explore special topics which are frequently difficult for men to talk about, such as dependency, homosexuality, and concerns about gender identity. The open acknowledgment of such topics within a group of men may serve to diminish the men's concern about these areas and to reinforce a greater openness in sharing a wider range of other feelings as well.
6. Men's groups may lead to a greater understanding of special problems for men, such as male diseases, an excessive need to achieve, reactions to divorce, and difficulties in parenting. The opportunity to hear about other men's experiences in these areas may be particularly helpful.

7. Men's groups can serve to alter the nature of adult male-male relationships by promoting caring and friendship between men.

8. Men may learn new patterns of relating to women in a men's group. The relatedness between changes in men and women is a recurrent theme for most men's groups, and relationships with women may be the central focus of some men's groups. Regardless of the extent to which the group explicitly discusses relationships with women, however, these relationships can be expected to be affected because the men are changing their ideas about themselves as men.

9. Men's groups can serve to increase the social and political awareness of men as a basis for eliminating individual and institutional sexism. Some men's groups are organized for the specific purpose of promoting radical change in existing gender arrangements. All men's groups, by encouraging awareness of gender role characteristics for both men and women, can help to increase the sensitivity of men to prejudices and injustices in society related to sexism.

## CHARACTERISTICS OF MEN'S GROUPS

Small groups of men have been shown to have characteristics which are different from the characteristics of women's groups and mixed groups. Aries demonstrated differences in these three types of groups which she believes reflect the sex role demands of conventional society (Aries, 1976). She showed that: ". . .men had more personal orientation in a mixed setting, addressed individuals more often, spoke more about themselves and their feelings, while in an all-male setting they were more concerned with the expression of competition and status." She also demonstrated that over time in a small discussion group men tend to benefit more from a mixed setting and women tend to feel less restricted and benefit more from an all-female setting.

Several other authors have also reported on specific problems in men's groups. Farrell extensively examines some major barriers to successful interaction in men's consciousness-raising groups which derive from the very conception of the masculine role in American society (Farrell, 1975b). One such barrier is the tendency of men to intellectualize. Through this process, men may become psychologically insightful or politically aware at an intellectual level without really changing underlying attitudes, beliefs, and behaviors. Another barrier to which Farrell refers is an inability of men to overcome their attachment to a hierarchy of values which places males' values over females' values in a social interaction. He believes that the maintenance of attachment to males' values leads to the development of such interactive traits as dominating, interrupting, condescending, showing disrespect, and aggression, traits which can interfere with showing empathy and warmth in interacting with others.

Washington (1979) identifies several problems for men in consciousness-raising groups. He describes the initial decision to participate in such a group and a sustained willingness to continue to attend as the two major problems to be overcome by such groups. Other problems he identifies include anxiety about homosexuality within the group and a tendency for the men to use intellectualization.

My own experience shows that for most men's groups these factors, when they are examined and when they are successfully managed within the group, may also provide a stimulus for further personal growth for the individual men in the group. Breaking through barriers to communication which present themselves as masculine patterns of relating to other persons appears to be the most satisfying experience reported by the men who have participated in men's groups. Certain specific features of men's groups, including the nature of the contract, the process, the pattern of leadership, the dynamics, and the presence of conflicts about changes will significantly influence the degree to which a particular men's group will successfully overcome the problems men have in interacting in small groups. I will now discuss two of these features, pattern of leadership and conflicts about change in more detail.

*Patterns of leadership.* Leadership is an extremely important variable in men's groups. Participants and observers in these groups agree that competition for dominance is an almost universal phenomenon in groups of men. The dilemma for most men's groups, if they recognize this struggle, is to establish a balance between some leadership, which can provide consistent direction and facilitation for group exchange, and non-adherence to traditional patterns of leadership, which are often directive, prescriptive, or authoritarian. Farrell (1974b) believes that men's groups need a facilitator initially to overcome males' inhibitions to group interaction, but that he should play a diminishing role over time.

The original purpose of the group will influence the pattern of leadership to some extent. If the group is formed for purposes of psychotherapy or education, then a therapist or instructor will usually serve as a leader. In contrast, if the group is constituted specifically for consciousness-raising or political action purposes, then leadership patterns may vary considerably. Some groups may rotate leadership, others may agree that there is no established leader, and yet other groups may use a set structure, such as a topic-discussion format, which addresses leadership by selecting a discussion leader.

Style of leadership is also an important issue for a men's group, regardless of how the leadership function is structured in the group. Moreland (1976) has emphasized the need for group facilitators in college classes about sex-role issues to be aware themselves about sex role constrictions and to model non-traditional patterns of behavior. It is difficult to imagine the members of a men's group achieving a higher level of awareness about sex-role issues and changing themselves if they were to be led by a person demonstrating only traditional sex-role attitudes or behaviors. Female leaders have apparently not been extensively used in men's groups, but this approach may provide an alternative for some men's groups which could both demonstrate that women can be in helpful positions of leadership in relation to men and at the same time provide for men a realistic representation of feminine qualities within an otherwise all male group.

If a group decides to establish itself without a designated leader or facilitator, it may encounter problems which can result in dissolution of the group, stagnation within the group or, if successfully handled, an enhanced sense of accomplishment by the group. The risks of conducting a men's group without a designated pattern of leadership are that the group members may persist in openly competing for leadership throughout the life of the group, thereby reinforcing traditional patterns of male-male interaction, or that the members may deny that competition exists at all. The latter outcome may serve to encourage even more unconscious mechanisms for achieving dominance through the use of intellectualization or reaction formation. Groups which can successfully overcome these problems without adhering to traditional forms of leadership may serve as the best laboratories for expanding male consciousness. Leaderless men's groups which cannot overcome these problems can benefit from using alternative strategies for leadership, such as requesting help from outside consultants or temporarily designating a leader from within the group.

*Conflicts about change.* Three specific conflicts regarding change often present themselves in men's groups and are a reflection of certain themes with which men in general are concerned today. These conflicts involve struggling with ambivalence about change, establishing a positive image as a man which incorporates both masculine and feminine traits, and resolving guilt associated with being a man. The members of a men's group must arrive at a motivation to change which is stronger than the motivation to maintain the *status quo* of gender role arrangements. The evidence that men suffer as men in our society is overwhelming. Goldberg (1976) has documented many of the negative aspects of being a man in America today, including a shorter life span than women, a higher crime rate, greater victimization as a result of crimes, and a higher incidence of many chronic diseases. But because men in fact continue to be in positions of dominance, continue to possess economic, educational, and political power, and continue to exercise prerogatives not available to women, giving up an association with the traditional masculine gender role is unacceptable to many men. Even if men, as individuals, derive little actual gain from the masculine role, they still have an association with power simply by being men.

A second conflict with which men's groups must struggle in order to allow change is to establish a more integrated sense of masculinity which does not deny traditionally "feminine" traits. Chodorow (1978) has stated that the masculine identity is to a large extent the result of a process which encourages boys not to be like their mothers. Many men, as a result, fear becoming like women if they acknowledge certain characteristics, such as the wish to be nurturing, passive, and dependent or the desire to possess other attributes traditionally associated with women. But to learn new ways of being men may be impossible for some men until they have first acknowledged their fears of being like women. The fear may be expressed in groups as anxiety about homosexuality or concern about being a "sissy" but it derives from an underlying devaluation of certain feminine-identified qualities.

A third conflict in some men's groups involves the personal guilt which men may tend to assume as a result of criticism of the masculine role. Criticism of the masculine role by some feminists and dissatisfactions with men expressed by individual women can lead to a personal sense of guilt on the part of some men simply because they are men. This guilt, if excessive, may prevent a group of men from freely examining what actual responsibility they have in their lives for oppressing women and ultimately from arriving at new definitions of masculinity which are associated neither with guilt nor with oppression.

## Application of Men's Groups in the Mental Health Field

Men's groups have not been extensively used up to this point either as an approach to counseling and psychotherapy or as a method of educating mental health professionals (Stein, 1982). Several reasons other than the fact that men's groups are not a widespread phenomenon in American society in general can be suggested for this paucity of experience. First, these groups can be difficult to work with because of the problems with competition and aggression which men present when communicating in small groups.

A second reason for the small number of men's groups in the mental health field derives from the fact that working with such groups may confront the leader with the same conflicts with which the men in the group must struggle. These conflicts include ambivalence about changing gender-role arrangements, difficulty in arriving at new expressions of masculinity, and guilt (for the male leader) about being a man.

Other reasons for the small number of men's groups in the mental health field include a general unfamiliarity with and lack of information about this approach to working with clients, a smaller number of men than women who seek psychotherapy and who are therefore available for participating in men's psychotherapy groups, and an absence of specific evidence regarding the effectiveness of men's groups in helping men who are in distress.

## The Applications of Men's Consciousness-Raising Groups

Men's consciousness-raising groups can serve to increase the awareness of men about problems arising as a result of enacting rigid, stereotyped gender-role expectations, to offer support for men who are sharing similar concerns in these areas, and to promote change among these men. These groups can be a valuable community resource to which men who present to psychotherapists or other mental health workers with such concerns can be referred in the same manner in which patients are referred to other community "self-help" groups.

Three examples where a recommendation to participate in an men's consciousness-raising group could be viewed as part of a comprehensive treatment and care program for men are with the substance abuser, the cardiac patient, and the man who is diagnosed as having one of the broad categories of disturbance classified as reactive or adjustment disorder associated with depression. These categories of problems represent characteristics which are related to the very definition of the masculine gender role. Specifically, each of these problems involves, in addition to many identified and hypothesized biologic factors, particular patterns of reacting to and coping with stress in the environment. The male alcoholic who reacts to anxiety by drinking; the compulsive, driven man who develops hypertension or has a heart attack; and the man who reacts to divorce with symptoms of severe depression can all be viewed as men who are in part enacting aspects of the stereotypic masculine role in American society. Through hiding feelings, through behaving in an excessively competitive and aggressive manner, or through viewing the loss of a relationship with a woman as a cause for lowering self-esteem and helplessness, these men may be enacting pathological extremes of the masculine role.

A second application of men's consciousness-raising groups within the mental health field is their direct use in the training of mental health professionals. Participation in a men's consciousness-raising group could accomplish the goal of increasing the individual male mental health practitioner's self-awareness regarding gender-role issues. Mental health training and continuing education programs have until this time generally failed to pay attention to the gender-related issues and sexism among men. Reports about the usefulness of women's groups for female trainees (Benedek, 1980; Kirkpatrick, 1975) suggest that there may be benefits derived from utilizing parallel groups for men as well.

## The Applications of Men's Psychotherapy Groups

The clinical applications for men's psychotherapy groups discussed in this section remain, at this point, suggestions for use, since little evidence exists that such groups have been widely used within the mental health field. Two principles must be considered if these applications are to become viable therapeutic alternatives. First, the same requirements which exist for evaluating the appropriateness of an individual for any psychotherapy group must also be applied in selecting men for participation in a men's psychotherapy group. Consideration is given to the setting and purpose of the group, the degree to which an individual man could benefit from participating in group psychotherapy, and the composition of a particular group. A second principle which must be applied is that men's psychotherapy groups must be studied as they are tried so that we can be more precise in predicting their usefulness for individual men.

Men's psychotherapy groups may be the desired treatment of choice for three types of men who are evaluated to be otherwise appropriate for group psychotherapy. These three types of patients are those with significant disturbance in interpersonal relationships, those with concerns about gender identity, and those men with specific concerns related to gender-role performance. These categories of patients may present with a wide variety of specific diagnoses and individual concerns.

No consistent criteria for selecting those men who could benefit most from men's psychotherapy groups can be presented. A helpful approach to selecting men for a men's psychotherapy group will involve assessment of the same areas which are evaluated in all patients combined with a particular emphasis on deciding how an all-male setting might be appropriate for an individual patient. For example, in obtaining a developmental history, specific developmental lags which are identified, such as failure to develop a relationship with father or failure to establish meaningful same-sex friendships during latency, may be reflected in current problems in interpersonal relationships. And men who are experiencing similar current life situations, such as divorce or job difficulties, may find a men's psychotherapy group particularly useful.

Men with a variety of physical diseases may also find a men's psychotherapy group helpful because this type of group will provide an opportunity to discuss those aspects of the disease which are associated with being a male in American society. The masculine gender role is especially relevant in considering two aspects of physical disease: first, the hypothesized relationship between the etiology of a variety of diseases, such as hypertention and heart disease, and patterns of coping with stress; second, the impact of physical incapacitation on the ability of men to function as males are generally expected to perform in our society. An excessive requirement for men to achieve and compete may contribute to the development of stress and associated physical diseases in some men. And the real or perceived loss of this same ability to achieve and compete which may be associated with certain illnesses for other men may lead to distress in the area of masculine identity. Thus, both the causes and the effects of physical illness may for some men be related to their experience of the masculine gender role.

The types of groups which would be appropriate for such men would depend on the degree of associated psychopathology and distress. Many men's groups which might be formed in general medical settings would probably not be designated as psychotherapy groups, but rather discussion groups. These groups might focus on reactions to loss, such as the loss of sexual functioning or of the ability to work. The important difference between these groups and groups of men which already exist in medical settings would be the focus on issues of gender-role expression and the relevance of these issues to the illness. For example, groups of male cardiac patients who presently meet for purposes of regular exercise and education could also be structured to encourage discussion of losses associated with the experience of being men.

A final application of men's psychotherapy groups might be within institutions, such as military hospitals and prisons, which are almost exclusively all male. Identified psychiatric populations within these institutions who are also evaluated to be appropriate for group psychotherapy could benefit from participation in a men's psychotherapy group. In some all-male institutional settings, such as prisons, there may be an increased likelihood that the environment will reinforce the development of particularly destructive expressions of the masculine gender role, including violence and excessive regimentation. In other all-male settings, within institutions particularly, concerns related to the experience of being a man may occur; such as homophobia or anxiety concerning athletic performance.

## EXPERIENCES AS A LEADER IN MEN'S GROUPS

Generally I conduct groups with a combination of the group-as-a-whole approach described by Bion (1961) and approaches emphasizing individual dynamics and interpersonal interactions. The style of leadership which I attempt to follow also represents some of the same characteristics which the men in the groups are seeking to acquire. For example, I present many of my interventions, which may derive from an awareness of unconscious and dynamic processes in groups and individuals, primarily as *alternative* insights. Thus, I attempt to listen without using what Farrell (1974b) labels as the masculine technique of self-listening. Some group leaders may believe that their explanation of a person's experience is the only correct understanding, and they therefore listen only in order to state their own insights and values about the experiences which group members relate. In contrast, I believe the leader in a men's group should more frequently demonstrate that he can simply listen to a group member and be able to admit the inappropriateness of an interpretation after discussion in the group.

Another example of a behavior which has altered because of my experiences in men's groups has been the degree to which I present intellectual in contrast to affective interventions in men's psychotherapy groups. Because many men have difficulty showing feelings directly, encouragement of the greater expressions of feelings may over time be more helpful for men even when an intellectual insight appears to be more appropriate or obviously relevant. I also frequently use self-disclosure regarding my immediate feelings in order to model the expression of feelings for men.

## SUMMARY

The future relevance of men's group for men in general will depend on many factors including the interest, motivation and capacity of individual men to function within small group settings. The greater utilization of men's groups can provide many men with the opportunity for an enhanced appreciation of themselves as men and for greater satisfaction in their relationships with other men and with women. The wider application of men's groups in the training of male mental health professionals can also lead to an increased awareness about the gender role concerns of practitioners and eventually of the clients with whom they work.

For some men traditional masculine activities such as athletic events and club or lodge meetings are being supplemented or even replaced by participation in men's consciousness-raising, support, or psychotherapy groups. The purposes of this article are to describe this occurrence as it relates to a growing number of men's lives and to encourage an increased application of men's groups in the future. The ultimate usefulness of men's groups will depend on continued and careful study of the benefits such groups provide to the men who participate in them.

# REFERENCES

Aries, E. Interaction patterns and themes of male, female and mixed groups. *Small Group Behavior,* 1976, *7,* 7-18.

Bion, W. R. *Experiences in Groups.* New York: Basic Books, 1961.

Benedek, E. P. and Poznanski, E. Career choice for the woman psychiatric resident. *American Journal of Psychiatry,* 1980, *137,* 301-305.

Bradley, M., Danchick, L., Fager, M. and Wodetzki, T. *Unbecoming Men.* Albion, California: Times Change Press, 1971.

Chodorow, N. *The Reproduction of Mothering.* Berkeley: University of California Press, 1978.

Farrell, W. *The Liberated Man.* New York: Random House, 1974a.

Farrell, W. Women's and men's liberation groups. In J. Jaquette (ed.), *Women in Politics,* Wiley, 171-199, 1974b.

Fasteau, M. *The Male Machine.* New York: McGraw-Hill, 1974.

Goldberg, H. *The Hazards of Being Male.* New York: New American Library, 1976.

Kirkpatrick, M. A report on a consciousness-raising group for women psychiatrists. Journal of the American Medical Association, 1975, *30,* 5.

Miller, J. B. Anger and aggression in women and men. Presented at the Annual Meeting of the American Academy of Psychoanalysis, New York, New York, December 2, 1979.

Moreland, J. A humanistic approach to facilitating college students learning about sex roles. *Counseling Psychologist,* 1976, *6,* 61-64.

Pleck, E. and Pleck, J. *The American Man.* New Jersey: Prentice-Hall, 1980.

Stein, T. The effects of the women's movement on men: A therapists view. Presented at the Annual Meeting of the American Psychiatric Association, Chicago, Illinois, May 1979.

Stein, T. Men's groups. In N. Levy and K. Solomon (eds.), *Men in Transition: Changing Male Roles, Theory and Therapy.* Plenum Publishing Corporation, 273-307, 1982.

Tolson, A. *The Limits of Masculinity.* New York: Harper & Row, 1977.

Washington, C. Men counseling men: Redefining the male machine. *Personnel Guidance Journal,* 1979, *57,* 462-463.

Wong, M. Males in transition and the self-help group. *Counseling Psychologist,* 1978, *7,* 46-50.

# Searching for the Hairy Man

Jack Kaufman
Richard L. Timmers

**ABSTRACT.** This paper reports on the use of a small group to assist men in a search for the maleness within themselves independent of the social expectations of male gender roles. The group was composed of male, helping professionals who saw themselves as responsive to feminism, believed they had begun to own and integrate their feminine aspects, but felt that something was still missing. Issues central to this search are presented.

## *Introduction*

We present, herein, an account of our experience with a group of men in which we sought to understand men better as well as ourselves as men. We shall describe what stimulated us, the plans we made, and what transpired within the group. Finally, we share the learnings and conclusions which grew from our experience. We believe a journey is as important as its destination. Our approach then is to reach beyond our intellect and to allow you into a part of our lives.

Historically, the male has changed considerably in the past thirty years. Back then there was a person we would call the '50's male, who was hard-working, responsible, fairly well disciplined: he didn't see women's souls very well, though he looked at their bodies a lot. . .then, during the '60's another

Jack Kaufman is Associate Director of the Wisconsin Institute, 106 East Doty Street, Madison, WI 53703. Richard L. Timmers is founder of the Midwest Sexual Counseling and Psychotherapy Center and a member of the Clinical Faculty of the School of Social Work, University of Wisconsin-Madison.

*163*

sort of male appeared. . .as men began to look at women and at their concerns, some men began to see their own feminine side and pay attention to it. . .Now, there's something wonderful about all this—the step of the male bringing forth his own feminine consciousness is an important one—and yet I have the sense there is something wrong. The male in the past twenty years has become more thoughtful, more gentle. But by this process he has *not* become more free. . .Many of these men are unhappy. There's not much energy in them. . .But now that so many men are getting in touch with their feminine side, we're ready to start *seeing* the wildman and to put its powerful, dark energy to use. (Interview with Robert Bly, Thompson, 1982)

Bly retells the Grimm Brothers' story of Iron Hans (Grimm & Grimm, 1977). The central figures in the tale are Hans, the wild, *hairy man* discovered at the bottom of a forest pond and caged, and the little boy whose precious golden ball subsequently rolls into Hans' cage. We believe the *hairy man,* a male energy or driving force, is a part of us which, for a variety of social and personal reasons, has been denied, suppressed, or distorted. We view the *golden ball* as a sense of radiant wholeness.

## Reflections

Robert Bly sang to us. The melody was familiar; we'd been singing it for some time. Not quite in awareness, uncertain of the words but, yes, he's singing our song! We were aroused and motivated.

Who or what is this wildman? Is he a part of us? Why is he hairy? Why is he in a cage? Who put him there? How have we kept him there? How do we set him free? Can we control him? Is this how we can get back our *golden ball?* What might happen to us?

We need help. Are others also experiencing these feelings? Can we call them together? Can a group of us look at what we have caged? If we put this part of us in a cage—can we let it out? We're going to have to think about nature/nurture again. Damn, is that never resolved? What is male about us? Have we lost track of it?

And so we embarked upon a quest to discover our own wildman and to learn to be guides for other questing men. This is a hard job! We don't know the territory ourselves, so how do we lead? We want men on this journey who will help and who will share the leadership. We want them to be friendly, compatible and good traveling companions.

## Preliminary Considerations

We believe that the rediscovery and integration of the wildman is necessary for men to regain the *golden ball* of wholeness and energy. We recognize that the social ferment of the last twenty-five years, the civil rights, anti-war, and women's liberation movements, has shaken many of our beliefs and assumptions about the nature of maleness. We have experienced, and learned from ourselves and our clients, that the discovery of our feminine aspects has changed us. We have recognized new vistas and possibilities. We have also experienced a loss, a feeling of void within. We are not always sure how to be male and energetic without being dominant and using our power to control others.

As social workers we have provided leadership in developing group work services for support and consciousness raising as well as problem-solving. In an effort to continue this pursuit, we invited a group of male professional peers to rediscover the *hairy man* and to explore and experience the nature of the *golden ball*. In a sense this exploration may be termed ''unconsciousness raising.'' We wanted to explore the subject *and* to learn how, through the small group process, to help other men find their inner male energy.

An informal written invitation and a copy of the Bly interview was sent to four men. We assumed that they would decline the invitation if they failed to reply. After each agreed to join the group, he received a fourteen-item questionnaire which we had developed. The questions were designed to explore parental influence before and after the age of eighteen; peer and friendship groups; a definition of macho and a personal statement regarding machismo and oneself; previous consciousness raising experiences; whether or not one described oneself as a feminist; the feminine and masculine parts of oneself; and a description of the composition of one's *golden ball*. The purpose of this instrument was to motivate and prepare participants to engage in the group task.

The group included four members with advanced degrees in social work and two with advanced degrees in clinical psychology. Ages ranged from thirty to fifty-one. Five were in long term marriages and one in a committed heterosexual relatonship. All saw themselves as supporting a sex-fair society. All believed they rejected "macho" values and recognized the need for a smorgasbord of gender roles.

## Charting the Course

The authors met weekly to review the prior session and to plan the next one. The group met for 9 sessions, described below. The narration organizes the sessions into three stages: beginnings, transitions, and recharting the route.

## Beginnings: Sessions 1-3

The questionnaire topics provided a basis for group members to begin their explorations of the *hairy man*. The initial session focused on those questions which dealt with our historical experiences. While there was a stated format for this session, members insisted they would decide *how* they would share their responses. While personal history reportings were basically information sharing about ourselves, the questionnaire items related to our awareness of masculinity/femininity within ourselves proved to be more difficult to capture and express. There was a reluctance to deal with one's own violence or violent impulses. This side of us tended to be suppressed or masked in issues of power and control. Intellectual explorations about power, control, and sacrifices in coupling dominated the discussion. The emotional aspects of these issues eluded us consistently, as if we were fearful to take ownership of the affective side of ourselves, to identify these feelings, and to share them openly.

A spirit of liberation emerged as we discussed the part of the questionnaire relating to the composition and location of our *golden ball*. The concept of the *golden ball* was familiar to all members and all believed it was something they owned at one time. Interestingly most identified it in terms of feelings and behaviors of the latency period. Expressions of a sense of wonder, enthusiasm and optimism, high energy, expressiveness, and physical contact emerged.

It was as if telling about these thoughts and feelings made the *golden ball* real and within our grasp. As the discussion continued, there was a gradual retreat from this affective side of us to emotionally distant discussions of abstract ideas. It seems to us characteristic of well-socialized males to avoid sustained emotion and we saw this as an example of caging the *hairy man*. The movement toward acknowledgement of the *golden ball* seemed too powerful to sustain and claim as masculine province. These qualities were debated as to whether they were masculine or human, and the relationship between biology and behavior neutralized the definition we had experienced. The reactions to this session however were a turning point in the group process.

## Transitions: Sessions 4-6

The next session started with the group members criticizing the abstract discussion of the previous week. They expresed a desire for more intimate involvement. Through the use of a guided fantasy which we developed, "Searching the Pool" (Timmers & Kaufman, 1982), we began to explore the resistances to confronting the *hairy man* within us.

The fantasy invited us to find ourselves alone in a primal forest, nude before a dark pool, within which was "something familiar." We were guided into the pool and given time and permission to explore its depths. A variety of symbolic images took form: a beautiful female guide, the creature from the Black Lagoon, an obstacle course of distractions, a re-birthing, and a primitive, pulsing, infant sexuality. Within these fantasy materials there were representations of the elements of conflict or avoidance. Each wanted to find the "familiar something," but all found or created obstacles to reach "it."

Again we were confronted with the elusiveness of defining the nature of the pool and ourselves within its depths. We did experience the recognition, however, of the difficulty and resistances to confronting the *hairy man* within us—a major step forward. Group members also responded positively to the structure represented by planning and presenting the guided fantasy. They suggested that the group leaders assume a more active role in planning and directing the flow of the remaining sessions. We welcomed this opportunity and our fears of being assertive with our peers began to dissolve.

In order to further our exploration of the emotional responses, in the next session we used a tape recording of poetry related to man's relationship to man and the expression of passionate/compassionate feelings related to the self and others (see "Related Readings"). Two themes evoked the strongest responses and images. The readings related to father-son relationships stimulated feelings about being fathers and/or sons, and the yearning for a "positive" father in our lives. The yearning related to the nurturing father whose presence and support was needed and necessary, but somehow not fully felt and experienced. We agreed that men need male cheerleaders.

The second theme that overwhelmed and disturbed our reflections related to violence. The inner violence we had briefly touched upon in an earlier session now faced us. We pursued this in the next session by using a tape recording describing a rare incident in which violence done by women to men was described by Chernin (1981).

This tape provided the stimulus to express fears and disgust related to violence, and to acknowledge a reluctance to discuss its dimensions and personal consequences. Group members were clearly aware of how men victimize women. To increase empathy they were encouraged to explore whether or not they ever viewed themselves as victims. They were reluctant to give or take ownership of physically violent feelings or behaviors.

Group members became more comfortable in examining ways in which they thought women controlled and/or dominated them. Themes of expressed dominance and submission were related to the expression of sexual intimacy. Those who thought they were responsible for initiating sexual intimacy expressed resentment. They wanted to share the responsibility as well as the pleasure and to be wanted sexually as well as emotionally and intellectually. This discussion prompted group permission and encouragement to explore ways of representing one's needs and wants. This expression of support was experienced by some as positive fathering, or professional helping, and by others as peer support. In contrast to the earlier discussion of father-son relationships, where the expressions of longing for change in relations was acknowledged but not problem solved, heterosexual relations were seen as an arena where change could occur.

### Recharting the Route: Sessions 7-9

The last three sessions were the beginnings of the recharting of the route to discovery of the *hairy man* and the *golden ball* by returning to the theme of the barriers preventing our reclaiming of this elusive side of ourselves: a guided fantasy, "The Trap" (Bellinger, 1975), was used to experience the feeling of being a trapped animal, to examine the trap as a representation of how we stop ourselves, and to provide an opportunity to free ourselves. Symbolically, the trap fantasy represented for us the caged man. It evoked variety in the choice of animal, in the detailed visual imagery, and in the problem solving used to escape. It is interesting to note that socialization as boys and men fostered and emphasized active problem solving on escape aspects of the fantasy, rather than other elements. We consciously chose not to interpret individual choices, but rather to encourage reporting of reactions, and discussing the exercise.

A touch exercise was designed to help members concentrate on sensations while touching or being touched and to be able to begin to accept feelings without acting upon them. We felt this was another aspect in exploring and discovering ourselves; for it opened up the importance of touch in our lives, as well as our personal conflicts about touching and being touched by other men.

Our closing session brought a new charting of the *golden ball*. We invited the group to summarize with images and passion their descriptions of the *hairy man* within, what characterizes this maleness and what still prevents us from ownership of our *golden ball*. The tone of the discussion was spirited, argumentative, yet cooperative, rather than competitive. We discussed what each of us needed to do to continue the expression of ourselves and to join with others in its pursuit.

### Emergent Themes

Our group experience has confirmed Bly's suggestion, that in the process of responding to feminism, men experience both gains and losses. The gains have been in discovering and legitimizing those aspects of the self which have traditionally been labeled feminine, particularly openness, expressiveness, and nurturance. The losses which men are experiencing are in the areas of energy, initiative, and joy. We speculate that power and control have often been viewed as positive energy reinforcers and that their loss depletes energy. It seems to us that sharing power and control is a better alternative.

A respect for feminism requires a redefinition of traditional male-female values and behaviors. Most men, however, have yet to find new channels for the energy and power which defines their essence of masculinity. It is our belief that the developing awareness of our female aspects must be integrated with our maleness. Awareness and acceptance of these males aspects is a precondition for such integration to occur. Since "real" maleness has multiple definitions, we assumed for purposes of this group that:(1) there is a *hairy man,* defined as male energy or driving force, deep within each of us; (2) we have lost, suppressed or given away that energy; and (3) in order for us to own our *golden ball,* a positive oneness or wholeness with the self, we need to re-discover it, claim it and allow it to co-exist with the social self.

In our work with this group a number of issues arose which we believe to be landmarks in the search for the *hairy man*: (1) difficulties in establishing personal definitions of maleness; (2) ambivalence about this task; (3) confusion between energy and violence; (4) relationships with men; and (5) relationships with women. Each of these issues is discussed below.

*Defining maleness.* Despite the clear physical differences between men and women, it is difficulty, if not impossible, to arrive at a single definition of maleness. This group had particular difficulty in accepting the *golden ball* as something male. They preferred an image of people as androgynous and desired to define all positive traits as *human* rather than male or female. While this position probably has much philosophical validity, it tends to reject our own experience of ourselves as men.

We do not claim to know what is intrinsically male, but research on physical and biochemical differences as well as on behavioral variation between male and female infants gives some basis for the belief that there are intrinsic as well as socialized differences between the sexes. Our working hypothesis is that both men and women need to identify and distinguish those feelings and behaviors that are intrinsic to ourselves and those that are socially learned. We need to decide which combination to use in becoming a person. Although it seems impossible to separate the nature-nurture puzzle, we believe there is value in the search for what is biologically determined and how we will adapt our biological assets/deficits to socialize our behaviors (Komarovsky, 1976; Unger, 1979).

*Ambivalence.* The group members had considerable ambivalence about seeking out their *hairy men.* The positive aspect of the ambivalence was expressed by joining this expedition. The view of the *golden ball* as positive and the possibility of recapturing an energy and sense of wonder were clearly attractions. The group's aggregate attendance of ninety-four percent, despite busy professional lives, was an expression of this positive side of discovery.

The negative side of the ambivalence was expressed indirectly as avoidance or resistance. This took the forms of intellectual or rational discussion, criticism of the leaders, and unwillingness to contribute suggestions for group activities.

Based on this experience we think it is important to encourage earlier, direct expressions of group members' ambivalence about discovering the *hairy man,* rather than postponing discussion of these fears. It is possible that this is a function of the male social role: approaching a difficult task by expressing one's hope and optimism and suppressing and withholding one's fears.

*Energy and violence.* Many people are familiar with the story of the prince who has been changed by an evil spell into a frog and how he is restored to his princely form by the kiss of a princess. In the original Grimm Brothers' tale, *The Frog Prince,* the spell is lifted not by a kiss but by the princess hurling the frog against the wall in a fit of anger (Grimm & Grimm, 1977). This demonstrates how we alter legends to "fit" contemporary views. The contemporary view this reflects is one of confusion and fear about the connection of energy, power, and violence which can block men in the creative use of their energy.

Our invitation to explore the possible costs of re-owning their energy elicited a number of fears which had to do with violence, selfishness, and questions about how this would affect important relationships. The issue of violence was a particularly difficult one for this group to approach. Most group members felt strongly that they would not commit physical violence on anyone, but were concerned about hurting others psychologically. There was cognitive awareness that this was not a violent act; however, there remained a fear of the existence, strength and effect of violent feelings. It became apparent that some of us confuse strong energy with violence.

> In *The Odyssey,* Hermes instructs Odysseus. . .that he is to lift or show Circe his sword. It was difficult. . .to distinguish between showing the sword and hurting someone. . .showing a sword doesn't mean fighting; there can be something joyful in it. (Thompson, 1982)

### Relationships with Men

> Is it utterly ridiculous for a man thirty-five years old and
>   graying
> To sit in his father's lap and ask for a bike?

> Even if he needs one?
> Whom shall he ask if not his father?
> Daddy, darling daddy, please buy me a bicycle.
>
> (Field, 1963)

This quotation with its explicit yearning for a father's nurturing touched group members strongly and raised a set of complex questions about male-male relationships. While the group members' experiences with their own fathers varied greatly, all felt a need for continuing nurturance from men. The topic of fathering evoked a variety of conflicted responses: we want male nurturing but we don't want to ask for it; we fear that accepting nurturing from another male will put us in a one-down, dependent position; we are uncertain whether or not we can move flexibly between a nurtured position and a peer position.

Ideally, in the course of the life cycle, we move from the dependent position of a child into a peer relationship with the adults who raised us. In simpler societies the rite of initiation provided a mechanism for dealing with this transition. For contemporary men this transition is lacking and much male-male interaction has a competitive and/or avoidant tone. The frequency with which men report competition and avoidance in their relationships with important men, especially their fathers, is undeniable.

The question of male to male relationships and homophobia was discussed. This fear was recognized as often present, mild, but always worthy of "working through." Group members were *less* concerned about their own periodic homophobia than they were about other men's potential homophobic response to them when they reach out. They want to be close and intimate with men; yet most would exclude sexual intimacy from those relationships. Our clinical experiences indicate this group of men have less homophobic responses than other groups of men that we have seen.

## Relationships with Women

All the men in this group had primary relationships with women and saw their female partners as their best friends. Considerable hesitance was expressed in the course of the group about how these relationships might be affected by ownership of male energy. Among the concerns expressed were: (1) being in touch with one's own energy would be too selfish or too dominating; (2) strong male-

male relationships would take too much time away from primary male-female relationships; and (3) being in touch with one's male sexuality and representing it to women might be viewed as too aggressive.

While none of these questions were resolved in the group, the sharing of these concerns served to increase the group bond and provided the opportunity for members to support and nurture each other.

## Professional Considerations

Our goal was to guide an adventure of discovery, and to explore interior rather than exterior sites of menace and mystery. Struggling with group issues required a leadership style and group structure which we began to develop in the process of working with the group and with our own internal conflicts. We focus here more on what we learned than on the mistakes through which our learning occurred. We present briefly the conceptual model which we developed from this experience and discuss our ideas about group activity and leadership style appropriate to the model.

*The initiation model.* The concept of *initiation* provides a useful way to think about this type of group. *Initiations* are transitions or transformations. These rites involve the discovery of inner strengths, the mastery of skills, and the overcoming of obstacles. These tasks are transversed in the course of moving from one status to another, usually from childhood to adulthood or from apprenticeship to mastery.

*Initiations* are also a part of the human cycle and reveal the nature of our relationships and prescribe the mechanisms for change. Thus, we all start as novices, grow to peerhood through the process of initiation, and, finally become initiators. This group initiated its members into a deeper recognition and appreciation of maleness.

*The group activity.* In structuring the group activity we sought "process-oriented behavior" which springs from the on-going content of shared experiences rather than "role-oriented behavior" which springs from external norms and expectations (Forisha, 1978). Thus, the focus of group activity was on creating a common experience designed to promote discovery and growth.

The first task in any group is establishing commonality of purpose. This was done by distributing the Bly interview and further reinforced by the questionnaire. In retrospect the question regarding the *golden ball* proved to be the most important element in focusing the relevant discussion.

An initiation must be experienced, not just talked about. In working with this population of men, it seems imperative to us to minimize opportunities for abstract, intellectual discussion and to utilize a range of directly experiential exercises. Such experiences involve reaching for unconscious imagery, touching the emotions, and physical contact.

*Leadership style.* We noted in the narration of the group experience that we were not very directive early in the group and in the transition stage responded to the group's request for more structure and direction. Our lack of directiveness in the beginning was a function of our fear of being too bossy and controlling with a group of male peers, our uncertainty about the territory, and our wish to be participants as well as leaders.

Our initiation model requires strong leadership in structuring a group's activity. The group members have their own anxieties about where the group may take them. They seem to need the reassurance offered by leaders who take responsibility for guiding the quest. As a group proceeds, members can be expected to seek more control of the activity as well as to provide more of the nurturing functions with one another.

For other group workers who might question, as we did, their ability to guide in this area, we hope our experience will be instructive. Though the scenery is unfamiliar, the qualities of being a good guide are known to the skilled group worker. The co-leader approach was particularly helpful to us in dealing with our wish to be participants.

## SUMMARY

Contemporary men have a responsibility to respond to the critical analyses of feminism. As men, it is to our advantage to use this stimulus to rediscover and express aspects of ourselves which traditional gender role definitions have banned. At the same time we must re-establish contact with our basic male energy, the *hairy man* within us in order to attain our *golden ball.*

The group reported on here was composed of professional peers, but the themes dealt with are, we believe, relevant to most men who have been responsive to feminism. On the basis of the group experience reported here, we believe the initiation model provides a useful guide for working with men to re-contact the *hairy man*. It provides the opportunity to recognize and deal with our fears of the unknown, to experience other men in cooperative and nurturing rather than competitive ways, and to experiment with new ways of expressing our energy.

## REFERENCES

Bellinger, L. D. Personal communication, 1975.

Chernin, K. *The Obsession.* New York: Harper & Row, 1981.

Forisha, B. L. *Sex Roles and Personal Awareness.* Morristown, New Jersey: General Learning Press, 1978.

Grimm, J. and Grimm, W. K. Grimms' tales for old and young: The complete stories. In Ralph Mannheim, trans. Garden City, New York: Doubleday, 1977.

Komarovsky, M. *Dilemmas of Masculinity.* New York: W. W. Norton & Co., 1976.

Thompson, K. What do men want? An interview with Robert Bly. *New Age,* May, 1982, 30-51.

Timmers, R. & Kaufman, J. *Searching the Pool.* Unpublished manuscript, 1982.

Unger, R. K. *Female and Male.* New York: Harper & Row, 1979.

## RELATED READINGS

Bly, R. My father's wedding, 1924. In Robert Bly, *The Man in the Black Coat Turns.* NY: Dial Press, 1981.

Bly, R. Finding the father. In Jim Perlman (Ed.), Brothersongs: A Male Anthology of Poetry. Minneapolis, Minn.: Holy Cow! Press, 1979.

Field, E. A new cycle. In Edward Field, *Stand up, Friend, With Me.* NY: Grove Press, 1963.

Ginsberg, A. Howl, Part II. In Allen Ginsberg, *Howl and Other Poems.* San Francisco: City Lights Books, 1956.

Hughes, T. Two legends and crow blacker than ever. In Ted Hughes, *Crow.* NY: Harper & Row, 1971.

Levine, P. My Son and I. In Jim Perlman (Ed.), *Brothersongs.*

Prévert, J. Song In the Blood. In Jacques Prévert, *Paroles Prévert.* San Francisco: City Lights Books, 1958.

Roberts, G. Andrew talks to gulls, for my son. In Jim Perlman (Ed.), *Brothersongs: A Male Anthology of Poetry.*

# TREATMENT GROUPS
# FOR VIOLENT MEN:
# TWO APPROACHES

We present here two papers by different authors in which they describe their approaches to working with men who have violent relationships with the significant women in their lives. Both papers were presented together at the Fourth Annual Symposium on Social Work with Groups. Each approach was offered as part of a comprehensive service for families experiencing domestic violence. The "Toronto" model focused on an exploration of gender issues, psychosocial factors, and altering the situations that lead to violence. The "Windsor" model focused on reducing the emphasis on blame and on helping the men to take responsibility for their actions.

# A Toronto Model

## David W. Currie

The Family Service Association of Metropolitan Toronto initiated its group work program for violent men in September, 1980. This program is part of the Domestic Violence Project which has been in operation since 1978.

According to Harris and Sinclair (1981), service for violent men requires interventions aimed at their (1) social context; (2) psychosocial factors; (3) lack of resources. Five major psychosocial factors are: externalized blame, fears of dependency, rigid definitions of masculinity, poor impulse control, and low self esteem. In this paper, we shall describe a group work service incorporating these types of interventions and directed at these factors.

## PURPOSE OF GROUP

One of the primary difficulties in counseling such men is to overcome their reluctance to be involved. In order to accomplish this, we set up a group program as we believed this mode would be less threatening to such men as it offers an atmosphere of support and understanding and it reduces the men's isolation.

The group met weekly for a two hour session for nine weeks. The size of the group was limited to six to eight members and two co-leaders. The members were men who are or have been violent and abusive in their relationships with women. The purposes of the group were to help members take responsibility for their behavior, stop violent behavior, and learn non-violent ways of coping with relationships. In addition we sought through the groups to help the men enhance other aspects of their lives. Within these broad group goals, we also sought to help the men to establish individual goals.

David W. Currie is a senior social worker at the Family Service Association of Metropolitan Toronto.

*179*

We initiated this service with pre-group interviews. Among the questions we asked during that interview were how long the man had been married or in a significant relationship; what type of violence occurred in the relationship, how it was perceived and what was its history; was the man ever beaten or abused as a child by his parents? Did he ever witness violence between his parents or anyone else in his family? Was there any alcohol abuse in his family? What did he hope to achieve by attending the group?

The following summaries of group sessions combine material from two men's groups. The sessions are divided into three phases. Sessions one to three (the beginning phase); sessions four to seven (the middle phase); and sessions eight and nine (the termination phase). In the beginning phase, the leaders assumed a structured and active role. In the middle phase, the leader's role was less active, and in the termination phase, the leader's role was again a very active one.

## BEGINNING PHASE

In the first session, the leaders described the origins of the service for couples with violent relationships as well as the purposes of the group. Introductions were made and the men were asked to tell something about themselves. The information they offered related to their marriages, families, job, hobbies, and reasons for coming to the group. After this process, the workers helped the members to state individual goals.

The workers presented information and led a discussion on what violence is, its causes, why it is a problem, why it should be stopped, how it originates, and how it relates to male and female gender roles and socialization. A sense of trust and cohesion began to develop during this first meeting. Leaders sought to be non-offensive with regard to violence (no "put-downs") so as to enhance the trusting atmosphere. An attitude of acceptance of the men as people was conveyed.

"Challenging" began to take place after the first hour but only on a superficial level. There was much testing yet the men acknowledged that violence was a problem. However, acceptance of responsibility for the violence was externalized by many of them.

A commitment was made by all members at the end of the session to stop the violence during the time period of the group. The men agreed to provide their phone numbers to each other at the second meeting to be used whenever there was a crisis or buildup of the problem. This was the beginning of the creation of a support network within the group and also a demonstration that there can be a wider community of caring.

During the second session, we helped the men to begin to accept responsibility for their violent behavior by having them identify cues or signals that are present prior to, during, and after being violent. These were:

*Before violence cues:* Feeling hurt, angry, physically tight, frustrated; silence (pressure buildup); pushing; shouting degrading remarks, sarcasm, or threats.

*During violence cues:* Out of control; things happening fast; physical abuse; self abuse.

*After violence cues:* Loss of self respect; loss of respect for partner; loss of friends; outside interference; silence; guilt; shame; physical shaking; weakness, wish to cry; fear; confusion about what happened and why.

These three stages of violence move from connection with self (before violence) to disconnection with self (during violence), to reconnection with self (after violence). Because "disconnection" is at the out-of-control stage, attempts at alternative behaviors must be made before then. We believe that the disconnection that occurs at phase two facilitates the denial of the violence at a later time. This is especially true with respect to severe violent episodes when many men reported at least a partial memory lapse for such events. This discussion of "phases" of violence served to help the men to become more aware of pre-violence cues so that they can become more open at that time to consider alternative ways of behaving.

The men were then asked for their ideas with regard to possible alternatives to violence. Among their responses were: make a telephone call, go for a walk to cool down; do something different; use another physical outlet such as chores around the house; arrange a short or long term separation.

The second part of the evening involved an open discussion of the men's personal situations. The information generated during the first part of the evening was also used here. Some of the men gave examples of behavioral alternatives they had tried that did not involve violence. They, therefore, provided role models for the other members. The group was quite supportive and the men encouraged each other to openly discuss their lives.

The third part of the meeting consisted of an anger exercise. This consisted of completing, in writing, a series of sentences such as: "When I am angry with people, I usually feel. . ."; "Three things that make me angry are. . ."; and "The things I can do to express anger more constructively are. . ."; the men read their responses to each other and these were discussed.

During the third session, there was an attempt by the leaders to help the men to take more responsibility for their violence. This was accomplished by asking the question "Who is responsible for violence?" The responses were significant as the men described some of their internal states prior to the onset of violence. This led to a more personal description than in the previous session.

Most of the men stated that the violence was done by them but there still was some externalization of blame on their partners: "If she hadn't said what she said," or "She hit me first," or "She really put me down." Another question asked of the men was "What are the benefits of stopping the violence and looking at alternatives?" Two particularly significant responses were: (1) "Stopping violence will relieve pressure on me and, as a result create a longer life," and (2) "The result will be increased closeness and intimacy in my relationship."

Occasional refocusing by the leaders was required during the discussion. Other themes which emerged during this process were being too dependent on one's spouse and bring afraid of this; and "losing out" in discussions of even small things. This "losing out" was associated with a loss of control and self-esteem and this was very threatening. Issues regarding control and domination also emerged.

The latter part of the meeting consisted of a discussion of the roles of male-female and husband-wife. An attempt was made to examine attitudes and values by asking the men to list the qualities that they saw as associated with each role. Some of their responses were:

*Male*—stronger physically and emotionally, more responsible, job oriented, unemotional, jealous, initiator of sex, threatened, seeking comfort, comforter, worse temper, illogical, irrational, egotistical, expresses self physically.

*Female*—more responsible, concerned with their bodies, able to show emotions, power hungry, insecure, complacent, upwardly mobile, more aggressive, roles changing fast, more confused, frustrated, sex object, emotionally colder, sensitive, calmer, logical, illogical, cunning, verbally antagonistic.

As the group continued to generate responses, there were more placed on the female side than the male. There was more difficulty in generating descriptive terms for males!

Descriptive terms for husband and wife were then asked for. Among the responses were:

*Husband*—House repairs, major decisions, sex initiator, pressure, needs to feel special, wants comfort.

*Wife*—Home management, dishes, kids, cooking, washing clothes, birth control, passive in sex, needs to feel special.

The discussion of these lists helped the men to realize that many of these descriptions were contradictory. Our purpose in pointing this out was to show the men that personality qualities and role tasks are not specific to one sex. We also pointed out that many of these qualities are assigned rather than inherent. We sought to increase the flexibility with which the men viewed themselves as males and their partners as females. At this stage of the group the men were moving in a direction of being better able to analyze role behaviors. They also were becoming aware of deeper feelings of insecurity related to the changes that are taking place in male and female roles.

During this group session, much more confrontation took place among all members and between leaders and members than occurred previously. This helped create an atmosphere of trust and cohesion. The men were also beginning to internalize responsibility for their own behavior and to experience themselves as separate individuals.


## MIDDLE PHASE

During the fourth to eighth sessions, we imposed less structure on the group. The purpose of these sessions was to allow the men opportunity to talk about their own situations. This was a time to integrate some of the material that had been presented during the first phase.

During session four, a film "Men's Lives" was shown. This film examines both traditional and emerging sex roles. Discussion of the film centered around the impact of early life experiences on later behaviors. We discussed how people's values too often were limited to striving for better cars, homes, and jobs. The ill-effects of this type of striving were considered including personal stress and marriage and family relationship problems. The men were asked to consider in this light the benefits of role changes.

At this point, the group had a lengthy discussion of parent-child relationships. Some personal examples from the men of their attitudes toward child raising were elicited. This led to an examination of sexism in both parenting and couple relationships.

Session five consisted of a discussion of developing a satisfying relationship. Two questions that served to focus much of this discussion were: (1) What qualities or characteristics do you value in your relationship with your partner? and (2) Why do some marriages survive? Some of the responses regarding these questions were: Qualities valued—trust one's partner and one's self; seek equality; share expectations; respect differences; share feelings; argue constructively; support your partner's interests. Marriage survival— Sex life; shared interests; knowing each other before marriage; speaking openly and sharing feelings; freedom for each individual; commitment; sharing values; able to adapt to changes; growing together.

The purpose of asking these two questions was to help the men to generate their own ideas about themselves and their partners. These ideas were pertinent to the men's ability to establish an individual identity based, in part, on qualities that they find valuable in their partners that they wish to support.

In sessions six and seven, we discussed a topic that had been raised frequently in previous sessions: how do people function in a relationship in terms of dependence and independence. To facilitate this discussion, we drew the following diagram on the board:

*Dependence-Independence*

| | | | |
|---|---|---|---|
| 0 | 0 | Independent | Distance-No intimacy, no support, loneliness. |
| | 0 | Dependent | Immobilized, not independent, insecure, NEED. |
| | 00 | Interdependent | Awareness, closeness, variety, respect for difference, movement, self control, friendship, WANT. |

Most of the men thought they had lost much of their independence through their marriage. This assertion led to a discussion of "control"—control over one's life as compared to control over someone else's life. We pointed out that in relationships in which the partners were extremely dependent on each other, there seemed to be a loss of a sense of personal boundaries. The partner was experienced as an extension of one's self. Thus, attempts to control the partner's behavior may, in part, be an attempt to have control over one's own life.

## TERMINATION PHASE

In session eight, the leaders began the termination process by asking what differences the men noticed in their lives since the beginning of the group sessions. Among the responses were: "I see two sides of the problem now and compromise more"; "I have increased self-control"; "I am better able to help others"; "I am more relaxed and sociable"; "I have increased self awareness."

Several of the men also commented that they wondered what the corresponding woman's group was covering. The men said they found their partners to be quite angry after most, if not all, of the sessions. They also felt hurt that their partners would not discuss what they were experiencing in their group. The men saw this as a lost opportunity to communicate with their partners.

The leaders explained both group programs and related the contrasting experiences of the two groups to the Dependency Cycle concept (Symor, 1977). A chart of this cycle is as follows:

Dependency Cycle

Dependent——Counter-Dependent——Independent——Interdependent

| (victim) | (anger-blame) | (Accepting responsibility for one's self) | (living with partner) |

(The descriptive terms in the parentheses are those of this author.)

We told the men that we believe that women in abusive relationships tend to enter counseling at the "dependent" stage. Men in such relationships tend to enter counseling at the "counter-dependent" stage and then move to the dependent stage before progressing. The men seem to move through the stages at a faster rate than the women and the women tend to remain in the counter-dependent stage for a longer period of time than the men to resolve those feelings.

As the men began to understand the cycle, they drew upon this to develop a respect for their partner's different growth process. This increased their ability to cope with some of the frustration they experienced with their partners during this group experience.

At the end of the session, the men were asked their feelings about the group ending. There was a sense of loss because an important source of support for them was about to be removed. However, there was also a sense that they were better able to develop other support networks.

In session nine, the final session, we obtained written and oral feedback about the group and we completed the termination process. The written evaluation included such questions as:

—What aspects of the group experience were most helpful to you?
—What were least helpful?
—What would you have liked to get out of the group but did not?
—Would you have preferred more or less direction from the counselor?
—Did you think that the topics discussed in the group sessions were generally related to your own problems?

## CONCLUSIONS

We see the group as an effective mode of intervention in working with men who are violent in their relationships with women. We were able to experiment with a number of program elements to gather a great deal of information relevant to working in this problem area. Based on this, we arrived at four major conclusions about this type of work.

1. Individuation of self—This relates to the issue of dependency. The men saw their partners as extensions of themselves when they

first entered the group and as separate individuals by the ending. When one sees a partner as an extension of one's self, behavior that is different from what one thinks is right is seen as threatening. This creates insecurity and may lead to violence. As the men began to see themselves as individuals, separate in mind and in body from their partners, their sense of self increased along with more tolerance and respect for differences between themselves and their partners. One step taken by some members that enhanced this process was physically separating and living in a different location from the partner for a period of time.

2. Internalization of responsibility—Throughout the group sessions, the men continued to move from a position of externalization of blame for the violent behavior to one of internalization of responsibility for it. This process of taking responsibility for one's behavior appeared to be an important step toward cessation of violence. As this process evolved, the men seriously considered alternative methods for dealing with the problem. Subsequently, the men assumed more control for their behavior.

3. Consciousness raising—This last major process occurred as we discussed roles and stereotypes in relationships. The men examined their attitudes and values including sexist perspectives. As a result, they were able to understand the unhealthy and unfulfilling aspects of relationships when these are based in sexism.

We also noticed as the group proceeded the men's ability to appreciate and begin to practice flexibility in role behaviors. This process resulted in their reporting that they felt less anxious and threatened in their relationships. This process was encouraged further by occasions when their partners responded positively to their changes.

Our suggestions for conducting groups of this type in the future are:

1. We believe that an educational combined with a therapeutic approach is a useful one. An educational component offers the members an opportunity to learn about alternatives that are conducive to growth and change. The therapy component allows the men the opportunity to examine aspects of their own behavior in depth.

2. Use of a blackboard and handouts is worthwhile in that this helps to provide a concrete, visual reference for the topic under discussion. This helps to maintain focus as well as progression from one topic to another.

3. We believe groups should be larger than the ones we con-

ducted. When some men missed a session, the group was too small. We would have liked to have had at least six to eight members present at each meeting.

4. An improved system for reaching out to such men should be devised. As this is a category of member that is hard to engage, it is imperative to have widespread recruitment through such devices as newspaper articles and pamphlets as well as through other agencies in the community such as women's shelters, counseling agencies, court clinics, and the police. Involvement of these members was voluntary. Mandatory referrals through the justice system should also be considered.

5. A selection of reading materials relevant to the topics covered in the group and compatible to the values of the program should be made available to members.

6. A planned follow-up session approximately four months after the final session should be held to assess the longer term effects of the group intervention as well as to provide another source of support for members.

## REFERENCES

Geller, J. A. Reaching the battering husband, *Social Work with Groups,* 1978, *1,* 27-37.
Harris, S. & Sinclair, D., *Domestic violence project: A comprehensive model for intervention into the issue of domestic violence.* July 1981, unpublished report, pp. 11-14.
Northen, H., *Social Work with Groups.* New York: Columbia University Press, 1969, pp. 98-99.
Symor, N., The dependency cycle: Implications for theory therapy and social action. *Transactional Analysis Journal,* 7(1), 1977.

# A Windsor Model

Lola Beth Buckley
Donna Miller
Thomas A. Rolfe

This paper presents an approach to working with male batterers developed at Hiatus House, Inc. which opened July 12, 1976 to serve Windsor and Essex County in Ontario, Canada. In the spring of 1981, a review of programs for male batterers in other communities was conducted. We were particularly influenced by a group called *Emerge,* a men's counseling service for domestic violence located in Boston, Massachusetts, and we drew upon and revised their approach.

## PROGRAM PHILOSOPHY

The way in which one defines the problem of domestic violence has a great influence on what one's programmatic response will be. There are three commonly held perceptions about domestic violence. The first is that the battered woman is responsible for the violence. She is blamed for it as well as being perceived as a victim. The second is that the male is to blame. The third is that the couple is in a cyclical interaction in which one or both partners have often experienced violence within their families of origin.

We believe there is no value in blame. There is often an intergenerational transmission of family violent patterns; violence is a learned behavior. We originally believed that violence in the relationship must be seen as the man's problem and he must assume responsibility for change. We have learned that perceiving violence as solely the man's problem and conveying this attitude prevented

Lola Beth Buckley is an associate professor at the School of Social Work at the University of Windsor, Windsor, Ontario, Canada. Donna Miller is the Executive Director of Hiatus House and Thomas A. Rolfe is a social worker at Hiatus House in Windsor, Ontario, Canada.

some men who batter from receiving service and we have altered our views.

## GROUP MEMBERSHIP AND GROUND RULES

Membership in the group was limited to men who were either presently involved or had been previously involved in a violent relationship with their spouse or significant other. The group began with four men with an upper limit of six to eight. After this initial experience, we decided that six is an ideal number.

Early in the program, men were referred after their partners had spoken with a counselor although we requested that the man phone and indicate where he could be reached. Men also frequently phone Hiatus House seeking information with regard to the whereabouts of their partner and children. It has been our experience that the man's contact with the agency can result in a request for counseling. Prior to the program described in this paper, the only involvement with the male partner was in couple counseling.

We also found that confidentiality can at times hinder the change process. A group rule about confidentiality that states one cannot talk outside the group about events occurring in the group is sometimes perceived by clients to mean they cannot communicate with their partner about issues they have worked on in the group. We now stress that people can be helped to communicate with each other if they begin by referring to something within the group in which they were involved. An example of this is "I've been thinking a lot about this since Joe said about me in the group. . ." Stress is placed on the importance for the man to take responsibility for his behavior and he has a choice (both inside and outside of the group) as to with whom he will share personal information. He is free, therefore, to talk about *his* experience in the group outside of it but not about the experiences of other members.

The group location was not disclosed to non-group members and the location was also one where the men would not be recognized or identified as belonging to a "special" population.

We also explained that all sessions will be audio-taped. The reasons that were given for this were as follows: (1) some behaviors are outside our awareness and it can be important to retrieve our behavior at a later date in order to assume responsibility for it; (2) the group member may wish to listen to the tape following a session in which they had "worked"; and (3) the tape will be used to develop treatment plans and for the supervision of the group worker.

The group would meet for one-and-a-half to two hours depending on the size of the group. The group worker would start and end the group "on time."

### Intake and Contracting

The pre-group process begins when the man calls and asks that the group leader contact him. Since suicide is a possibility with some men in this situation, we return this call as soon as possible and never later than twenty-four hours. During this conversation we are sensitive to any indication that suicide is a potential such as how the man responds to the invitation to attend an interview. The subsequent individual assessment interview lasts approximately an hour unless suicide is still a concern. Group rules, such as those noted above, are explained to the man and an invitation is offered to attend introductory group sessions.

The basic purpose of the group, to stop abusive behavior, is identified as well as a number of additional goals that include learning alternate behaviors, learning to express anger in constructive ways, being able to identify feelings, learning better ways of communicating, acquiring problem-solving skills, learning new and more flexible attitudes toward women and identifying the roots of anger and violence in one's self and the impact of such behavior on others.

We emphasize that the potential of the group can best be realized if the men view it as an opportunity to both "get something" for themselves as well as help others. We also use an intake questionnaire to assess the men's motivation for the group although we explain the "answers" and assure them that the questionnaire will have no effect on group membership; even completing the form is optional.

## PROGRAM STRUCTURE

The group meets for eight weekly sessions. New members are introduced during the first two sessions only. The group may also contain men from previous groups who have contracted for additional sessions. (We contract initially for only eight sessions because we find that the men's motivation will support this commitment; the

group experience itself leads to an increase of many men's motivation to change.)

During introductory sessions the men tell what has brought them
to the group. The goals that will be worked on in the group are
developed in the second session. A written contract signed by each
member is finalized in these first sessions. It states that the men are
expected to attend group sessions on time. An important stipulation
is that if a member is absent from the group, the meeting is can-
celled. In the event a member is absent, the other members will contact him to ascertain whether he is having severe problems. The
reason for this requirement is to enhance the men's sense of responsibility for each other, an area in which many members have problems in all of their relationships.

Group members exchange phone numbers so they may seek support from each other in crisis situations. If a man expects to be absent from a meeting, it is his responsibility to call *all* the members
and inform them there will be no meeting.

The eighth session of the group consists of an evaluation. During
the first forty-five minutes of that session the man's significant other
is invited to give the man feedback on his progress. This person is
asked two questions: what changes has she noticed in the man and in
what ways does he still need to improve.

### First Sessions

Initially the members are uncertain about whether they can trust
the men in the group. They fear failure. They want to stop the
abusive behavior but are afraid they will not be able to succeed.
They have a desire to be close to others and they want acceptance; at
the same time they are afraid of being vulnerable and of being hurt.
In this early stage, members are unsure about how much to commit
themselves to the group. The purposes of the group are reviewed
and an agreement in the form of a contract is reached. Members also
discuss individual needs and establish individual goals.

### Middle Sessions

Ways are established to help members to meet their own needs
within the structure of the group. Members are likely to test the
worker and to look for proof of his caring and acceptance. Members
begin to express trust in other members and to express their feelings. They bring problems to the group and do so with less fear of

being rejected or punished. Cohesiveness develops as the men find that they can argue with and confront each other. The worker flexibly assumes different roles within the group; at times he is more and at other times less active.

The worker during this period sometimes confronts members about irrational thinking and unacceptable behavior. Toward the end of this stage of the group's development, the men begin to talk about changes they have made in their lives and the successes they are experiencing in dealing with their anger.

## Final Sessions

During the last two sessions the worker talks about termination. He encourages the men to talk about changes they have experienced in themselves and their relationships. The worker also points out what could happen to cause the men to return to abusive ways of behaving. The men are likely to acknowledge improvement while indicating they fear the loss of the group's support.

During the eighth session, an evaluation takes place. As we stated above, the men bring a partner. The criterion for whom they bring is that this person must be aware of their violence and must have sufficient contact with the man to acknowledge changes he has made. During this feedback session the rules are that only one person at a time may speak; the partner should direct comments to the man; the man may not interrupt the partner; and once the partner has finished the man may ask for feedback or clarification and then respond to that. If the group member has already indicated that he is going to continue in a group some homework may be given to the couple. Once each couple has ''had a turn'' the partner is asked to leave the session and the men continue with their group evaluation.

Some men deny that the group has had any influence on their behavior. Others regress to earlier patterns. A few chose ''flight'' as a way to end the group. Three men who were group members have enrolled in a training session to develop skills to work with men who are on the waiting list of the agency.

## CASE EXAMPLE

The member has been involved with the program for six months and is preparing for termination. At this time there was no longer any physical abuse in the relationship. The couple had separated at one time in order to "give each other space" as they thought that violence could reoccur. Since there were children involved, the man took responsibility to move out of the house rather than his partner or children, as is usually the case. This is a positive indication of progress.

Within the group the man had talked about being abused as a child. His current work in the group focused on his opinion of women and his view that women were "useless tits." He did not know how he had come to that opinion because he realized that a number of women including his partner were very competent.

During one session, the worker asked this member if he were willing to explore this view of women further and he agreed. The worker asked him to remember a time when he has being hit by his father. The event he recalled was when he was ten years old and his father had "taken a belt" to him. During that time, he recalled that he fell on the floor and tried to avoid the blows by assuming a fetal position. His father continued his attack.

The worker asked the member to assume the same fetal position on the floor. The worker took his belt off and acted as if he were hitting the man. At this point, the worker asked the man where his mother was. He stated she was standing in the corner crying. The worker asked him what he, as "that ten year old boy," wanted her to do and he stated he wanted her to make his father stop beating him.

At that point, the member realized that one reason he felt as he did toward women was that his mother was not able to stop his father from beating him and for him, as that ten year old boy, this was the most important thing she could have done. The man through this discussion came to the realization that his mother could not protect him without endangering herself even though she had provided this protection on several occasions and had been attacked. Following this episode, the man began to experience a change in his attitudes toward women.

## SUMMARY

In this paper, we have outlined the rationale for and the nature of a program of group services for violent men. We have concluded that many such men are open to this type of group experience and that they can make significant changes within a relatively short period. We have encouraged some men to re-enroll for an additional six sessions and this has also been valuable. Our approach is marked by a de-emphasis on blame together with a strong injunction that violent men take full responsibility for their destructive behavior.